Aloevera

Amazing Benefits of Aloe Vera Plus a Delicious

(A Complete Guide on Treatment of Diabetes Using Aloevera)

Louis Bigelow

D1108954

Published By **Elena Holly**

Louis Bigelow

Aloevera: Amazing Benefits of Aloe Vera Plus a Delicious (A Complete Guide on Treatment of Diabetes Using Aloevera)

ISBN   978-1-77485-751-9

No part of this guidebook shall be reproduced in any form without permission in writing from the publisher except in the case of brief quotations embodied in critical articles or reviews.

Legal & Disclaimer

The information contained in this ebook is not designed to replace or take the place of any form of medicine or professional medical advice. The information in this ebook has been provided for educational & entertainment purposes only.

The information contained in this book has been compiled from sources deemed reliable, and it is accurate to the best of the Author's knowledge; however, the Author cannot guarantee its accuracy and validity and cannot be held liable for any errors or omissions. Changes are periodically made to this book. You must consult your doctor or get professional medical advice before using any of the suggested remedies, techniques, or information in this book.

Upon using the information contained in this book, you agree to hold harmless the Author from and against any damages, costs, and expenses, including any legal fees potentially resulting from the application of any of the information provided by this guide. This disclaimer applies to any damages or injury caused by the use and application, whether directly or indirectly, of any advice or information presented, whether for breach of contract, tort, negligence, personal injury, criminal intent, or under any other cause of action.

You agree to accept all risks of using the information presented inside this book. You need to consult a professional medical practitioner in order to ensure you are both able and healthy enough to participate in this program.

TABLE OF CONTENTS

Introduction

Aloe Vera is always more than a marvellous plant. I am extremely eager to share the important details about this amazing herb with you. The reason I wrote the book was to share how to use aloe vera. It was used extensively by our ancestors to treat various problems like constipation, sunburn and rashes, wound healing infections, wound healing, etc. It will surprise you to find out that it is becoming increasingly popular in the present days , as scientific research has proven its effectiveness.

Aloe Vera is an ideal mixture of vitamins, proteins minerals and enzymes. It is a pleasure to find out that you can utilize it internally and externally with no adverse consequences. You can use it safely for your children as well. In this book you will also learn how to make use of it. The most appealing aspect of the herb, is that it's equally effective for conditions of your pets as well as other animals.

If you've never had the chance to be aware of aloe vera, then you're very fortunate to have a chance to read this book. This book will show you the incredible advantages of the aloe plant. It's an "all treatments" plant. I am certain that once you read this book you'll become an aloe vera, just as I am. You must be contemplating planting aloe vera plants in your garden so you could enjoy the many advantages of this organic medical herb.

What are you still Let's dive into the magical universe of the aloe plant, and be awed by it.

Chapter 1: Aloe Vera: A Miracle Plant

In truth, aloe vera is a wonderful gift from God for humans. The plant is an organic wonder plant. It has been utilized for centuries and is also a popular herb this day and age. The reason is its unique composition. The medical science community has proven its benefits in terms of health.

Before we move on into the benefits and uses we'll go over a brief overview of the aloe vera plant for your greater understanding.

About the Plant

Aloe Vera is an herb that is succulent. It is part of the onion family and Garlic, however its plant is distinct from the other. It is mainly found in warmer climates. It is a small-stemmed plant with fleshy, horny leaves. The plant is comprised of the three components:

1- Aloe vera roots:

The roots of aloe vera aren't so deep in the soil. Aloe vera's roots are more like strings and threads extend into the soil in the manner of an beetle. The tiny roots are able enough to supply nutrition and water for the plants.

2- Aloe Vera stem:

Aloe vera is a very short stems that are extremely short. It's so short it is frequently referred to as a non-stemmed plant. It's hard to tell. It appears to be leaves sprouting from roots. The stem is only visible after cutting its leaves near the base.

33 Aloe Vera leaf:

Leaves make up a large component of this plant. Its leaves are thick soft and hairy. Aloe vera leaves have three layers.

Its outer layer extremely hard and protects. It is responsible for the production of protein in the plant.It is somewhat bitter, however it is a good chemical for natural protection for animals.

* The middle layer contains anti-inflammatory, antibiotic, laxative and painkiller properties.

The innermost portion of the plant's the most soft and supple. Its main element is water that makes up the majority of it. Alongside that, vitamins, minerals, proteins and lipids can be found in trace amounts.

4Stalks and flowers:

In spring in the spring, a stem of aloe vera is spotted within the middle of the plant. The flowers are tubular which contain seeds. The seeds can be capable of transforming into a fully-grown plant.

Aloe vera is a component of the composition

Aloe vera comes as a blessing from God. It is perfect to its constituents. The main ingredient is water which accounts for nearly 90% of it. The remaining 1percent is composed of various nutrients. The nutrients include:

VITAMINS:

Aloe vera is a great source of vitamins. In this regard vitamins, vitamin C is on most prominent. Aloe vera also has Vitamin E that is good for skin and hair. It also has a tiny quantity of Vitamin A. Vitamin A is an antioxidant found in nature , and can help eliminate free radicals in the natural way.

Vitamin B12 and Folic acid are beneficial for digestion and gut health. digestion.

MINERALS:

Aloe vera has calcium and copper as well as iron, chromium magnesium, sodium and zinc. The majority of them are required by different enzymes for their proper function. A few are anti-oxidants.

SUGARS:

Aloe vera is a source of monosaccharides and polysaccharides. These sugars are natural anti-allergic as well as anti-inflammatory.

HORMONES:

It is a source of hormones that aid in the healing process and also reduce inflammation.

Amino acids:

Aloe vera is abundant in amino acids. Some of them are essential amino acids. They are the precursors for protein synthesis during healing. This helps reduce inflammation and encourages healing.

ENZYMES:

Aloe vera contains a variety of types of enzymes. Certain enzymes help are able to reduce skin inflammation. Other enzymes play a crucial role in the digestion of sugars and fats.

STEROIDS:

It provides steroids that are great to treat fever, inflammation and discomfort.

ANTHRAQUINONES:

They are also known as laxatives. They aid in protecting against bacteria, viruses and fungal infections. It also has anti-inflammatory the natural world.

Chapter 2: Internal Health Benefits Of Aloe Vera

Aloe vera can be beneficial in many ways.It can be utilized in a variety of ways both internally as well as externally. To use internally it is available as a salads, juices, or juices as well as dry form.

The first thing to remember when taking aloe vera internally is to always be aware regarding the dosage. Since it is a medicinal plant, as with all other medications, it must take a specified amount and in a certain intervals as recommended by experts. In excess, it could be harmful to your health , so be aware. We will go into detail the dosage of this product and its possible adverse effects in later chapters.

Let's take an overview of the benefits to your health from aloe vera in greater detail. Let's begin with

1Aloe vera, gut

Aloe vera is known for its help in digestion. It's effective in treating stomach problems. Constipation is the most common. The majority of research and studies have a positive view of the laxative aspect of constipation.

Treats Constipation:

Aloe vera has been renowned for its ability to laxify the body over the years. It's beneficial for the proper function of your digestive system. It also aids in cleansing the digestive tract.

In constipation, there's reduced bowel movements. Constipation is mainly caused by the absence of fiber and water in food. Aloe vera gel is high in water and other essential nutrients. aids in controlling the stool movement.

Aloe vera can be used in a safe way to ease constipation. It is extremely effective in preventing constipation. It generally takes only a couple of hours to achieve the desired outcomes.

Treats GERD:

Let's begin by letting me introduce you to GERD. It's a gastro-esophageal reflux disease. In this condition, the most prominent symptom is heartburn. Aloe vera juice is acidic and helps fight the acidity that causes heartburn.

You can also use aloe vera in order to treat heartburn and maldigestion.

Treats Diarrhea:

Aloe vera is also utilized to help treat diarrhea. Since aloe vera acts as an adaptogen. It aids in cleansing the intestines. Aloe vera helps in removing harmful bacteria from the digestive track, leaving only the beneficial flora. This method, it removes worms from the intestine.

It is therefore equally effective for constipation and diarrhea.

Healthy Weight loss:

Aloe vera can help people who wish to lose weight naturally. Through improving digestion, aloe vera is a secondary cause of weight loss. Because the bowel helps to reduce the burden of toxic substances and also energizes the body, weight gain is prevented. Additionally, it plays a role to reduce fats.

The great benefit of aloe vera is that it assists you appear more attractive, more fit and slim.

2-Boost the immune system

Aloe vera is a great way to boost your immune system and aid to work effectively. It is abundant in immune-boosting components and polysaccharides. Polysaccharides boost your white blood cells.

The white blood cell:

White blood cells constitute the essential component that make up our body's immune system. They are vital to defend our body. They fight off germs to shield our body from illness. Aloe vera's polysaccharides boost the creation of white blood cells. This makes our immune system stronger.

DETOXIFICATION:

Aloe vera also enhances the immune system by the help of its anti-oxidants.Anti-oxidants act by removing the free radicals (bi-product of various body reactions and hinder its normal functioning and contribute to aging process) from our body.

3 Good for respiratory problems.

You'll be happy to know that you may utilize aloe vera to treat respiratory problems too.

As the juice of aloe vera is rich in Vitamin C (ascorbic acid) which can be helpful in relieving symptoms of common cold, run nose, flu, cough, and so on.

It also contains magnesium lactate, which can be effective against allergic reactions . It is can also help with inflammations.

4-Fights against infections

Everybody in the world is prone to becoming infected at any time of life. The consumption of aloe vera can aid fight diseases. It is a great remedy for any kind of infection.

Aloe vera is unique by its chemical composition. It contains numerous active ingredients that work in a unique way to fight the organisms that cause illness. It assists in the treatment of infections caused by bacteria. It can also be efficient in treating fungal and viral diseases too.

Immune boost feature is another benefit to. It allows you to fight off germs to avoid diseases.

PRECAUTION:

If you have a history of chronic illnesses, do not try home cures. It is better to seek the advice of a physician and have the treatment you need according to the doctor's recommendations.

5-Treats for inflammations

It is renowned for its anti-inflammatory properties. It is extensively used to alleviate pain and inflammation during arthritis, which is the joint inflammation. It doesn't just ease the pain but also helps slow up the inflammation process dramatically.

You'll be shocked to discover that aloe Vera can reduces inflammation and aids in healing in the same way. If you consume aloe vera in your body, it will help treat any inflammation in your body.

6-Cardiovascular benefits

When taken internally, is great for the health of your heart. Many studies are in for it. You want to learn what it does to reduce the chance of cardiac arrest.

It works by reducing the level of cholesterol in the body . It also boosts the capacity of oxygen transporting the red blood cells. Aloe vera reduces the cholesterol levels by eliminating the excess cholesterol in the human body. It consequently regulating blood pressure as well as the oxidation process.

If you have a heart condition or have a strong family history then you must take aloe vera on an ongoing basis to protect the heart.

PRECAUTION:

Be aware of one thing, heart issues are typically life-threatening, so don't use home remedies as your sole source of. See a heart expert on a regular basis and talk to your doctor to prescribe Aloe vera.

Inattention to its use could result in a major issue. Therefore, it is essential to take care because the life of a person is precious.

7-Treat diabetes

Aloe vera is also beneficial for people suffering from diabetes. It assists in regulating the blood sugar levels. It's not just for treating diabetes, but can also help stop it from occurring if it is used regularly.

Diabetes can lead to serious issues when it becomes worse. Care must be taken. A person should consult with their physician prior to using aloe vera, and inquire if it is beneficial or not for their health. It could react with medications that control sugar or not?

It is only allowed to be used only if it has been declared to be safe by your physician.

8-Anti carcinogenic

The plant's miracle has anti-carcinogenic properties. It aids in fighting against cancer. It aids in reducing the size of tumors and promote the expansion of normal cells.

There is not much research done on the aloe vera plant in this way. Researchers are still working to prove the benefits of aloe vera.

9-Relieving stress

Stress is an integral element of our everyday lives. In everyday life, the majority of us get stressed and this is detrimental to our well-being. Also, aloe Vera will aid you in this respect.

The aloe vera juice is extremely refreshing. It helps improve blood circulation, which is not just beneficial for the health of your heart, but also assists in removing out fatigue and stress out of the body.

It is a great way to reduce stress. Drink it as a juice to reap the benefits. Aloe vera that is used in excess is not recommended. It is not advised to use regularly, but only every once in a week.

10Aloe vera, and the female reproductive system:

Aloe vera is a remedy for treating menstrual irregularities. It is most often utilized by single women. If you experience irregular menstrual flow you may use it but do not use it during menstrual cycles.

Aloe vera assists women in regulating her hormones. It helps to keep her young and healthy.

11- Aloe vera , and joints:

Osteoarthritis is the most frequent joint inflammation that is caused by age. With this type of condition joints can be extremely painful and swelling.

Aloe vera can be used for treating arthritis by decreasing inflammation. Its analgesic qualities help alleviate the pain. Aloe vera does not just reduce inflammation, but also helps to heal by supplying amino acids and vitamins.

Adult Dose that is safe for children:

Adult male (50-70 kg)... 1 Table spoon

Adult female (50-70 kg)..................................... 1 Table spoon

PRECAUTIONS:

1. Avoid using aloe vera juice to treat internal use on a daily basis.

2. Try it once per week, but not more than twice per week.

3. If aloe Vera does not cure a specific ailment, do not increase the dose.

4. It is recommended to see your physician for an expert opinion.

5. In excess, aloe vera can be harmful.

6. If you use aloe vera, one could become resistant to it.

Chapter 3: External Avoids To Health Of Vera

In the last chapter, we have talked about the internal health benefits of aloe vera, but now we will concentrate on its external advantages. It is much easier to utilize the herb externally rather than internally, since in external usage, there is no care needed. Another advantage of the external application for aloe vera, is the fact that it comes with zero adverse side effects.

Aloe vera has been proven to be effective in treating various skin issues. Due to its many advantages, this miraculous healing plant is also the primary ingredient in a lot of cosmetic products. Let's take a look at it.

1-Natural healer:

The plant is considered to be an amazing plant due to its therapeutic properties. It is beneficial in a variety of ways.

Treatments for sunburns

Aloe is able to treat sunburns with ease due to its strong treatment ability.As the gel of aloe is made up of 99 percent water, it aids to soothe the skin. It aids in healing through the aid of its nutrients and anti-oxidation qualities.

All you need do is remove the leaves of its gel and then apply to the skin that is affected. It provides an enveloping layer on the skin and aids in healing.

Useful for frostbite prevention:

Aloe vera is also utilized to heal the damage caused by frostbite by increasing blood flow to the affected region and enhancing the growth of cells near the location of injury.

God forbid and if you suffer frostbite, do not worry about it at all. Take aloe vera gel fresh from its leaves to apply an even layer to the area affected. Apply gentle pressure to the affected area for a few minutes.Repeat the process many times throughout the day. The area will improve each day. If your condition isn't improving,, then talk to your doctor for a professional advice.

The healing process:

Aloe vera is an effective home remedy to heal wounds. It can be beneficial for small cuts, healing scars as well as thermal burns. Numerous studies have also proven that it is effective for minor cuts, healing scars, and thermal burns.

In the beginning, it cleanses first of all it disinfects the Site that has been injured. The naturally occurring steroid found in these plant reduces inflammation. The cooling effect generated by the gel of aloe vera helps in the formation of new cells near the site of injury.

It can be used in cases where the wound isn't deep enough in the skin. If it's a severe type of injury, don't depend on your own solutions. Consult a doctor immediately before the condition gets any worse.

Aloe Vera to lips:

Aloe vera is useful for swollen lips. It can be used for dry lips too because it can help moisturize the skin, and repair the damage.

It is possible to apply aloe vera gel that has been freshly extracted from its leaves onto the area affected, and then massage gently for a couple of minutes, then let it dry. Repeat this procedure for a few days to achieve the desired outcomes.

It can effectively treat chapped and inflamed lips.

Allergies:

Also, you can apply aloe vera to treat various allergies. It is useful for those with sensitive skin. It can be quite helpful with the itchy skin that is common in-hand eczema. It also helps to get rid of it.

Utilize it on a daily schedule and you'll soon be able to see the effects.

Aloe vera is a great foot moisturizer.

Aloe vera is a great remedy for fungal infections. Soldiers and athletes are likely to have the feet infected. Aloe vera gel can be efficient in treating this problem.

Extract fresh aloe vera gel, and apply it on the skin affected on the area between toes. Apply gentle pressure to the area affected for a some minutes, then remove it. It could take between 3 and 4 days, depending on how severe the condition.

It is also employed for foot scrubs. It hydrates the skin and aids in the removal of the dead cells of skin.

Aloe vera for after shave:

Aloe vera is a popular ingredient for after shaving due to its soothing effects. It aids in moisturizing the skin and assists in healing the small cuts. Aloe vera can also be an vital ingredient in the various shaving gels for aftershave that are available on the market in their prepared form.

It is possible to use aloe vera gel aftershave to reenergize the skin and treat small cuts. Apply it right after having finished shaving. Massage gently and allow it to rest for a few minutes, then rinse it off with tap water.

It will be felt to your skin. It will feel extremely soft and silky.

2-Aloe vera and cosmetics:

Aloe vera is the top best natural secret to beauty that has been revealed to the world. It is the most important ingredient of almost all cosmetics due to its numerous benefits for the skin.

Aloe vera is gentle on skin, in all circumstances.

Enhances the appearance of skin:

Aloe vera is abundant in vital nutrients that are essential to maintain healthy and beautiful skin. It hydrates the skin, while also removing dead skin cells and encourages the development of cells. It also removes the pigments off the skin, making it radiant and fresh. Vitamin C and E play an significant roles as they neutralize free radical oxygen.

An incredibly thin coat of Aloe gel is sprayed on the neck and face. Apply it for about 15 minutes. It is possible to apply this to the skin on daily basis to eliminate spots and pigmentation. After that you'll be left with a smoother, more radiant and more flawless skin.

It is good for Acne:

Aloe vera is beneficial in oily skin. It can help treat pimples naturally , and can help remove the marks too. Pimples can be caused by bacteria, and aloe vera is beneficial for bacteria and helps to reduce hyperpigmentation thanks to the aid in vitamin C as well as vitamin E.

If you suffer from oily skin, then you should be extremely happy to learn about it. And you should have decided to try aloe vera as a remedy. Aloe vera gel can assist you in this way.

Use Aloe vera gel on your neck and face. Massage it for a few minutes and leave it on for about 10 to 15 minutes so that it absorb completely. Rinse with tap water. Pure aloe vera gel could be used in conjunction with it, or mix it with a fruit extracts of your choice to boost its effectiveness.

Apply aloe vera at least once every week, and maximum two times per week, but no more than the recommended amount.

Dry skin is moisturized:

If you're suffering from dry, flaky skin, don't lose the hope. Aloe vera is a must for everyone. It also benefits your skin. It can be used to nourish your skin, without making it oily, that's why it's also great for skin that is oily.

Aloe vera is rich in enzymes and vitamins that help to keep moisture into the skin. This results in healthy, radiant and beautiful skin.

Spread a small amount aloe vera, and massage it gently for a few minutes. It should remain for between 10 and 15 minutes. Rinse it off using tap water. It will be evident the effects after just one application. It is recommended to apply it one time per week.

Removes under eyes dark circles:

Dark circles under the eyes are typically caused by anxiety, sleeplessness and headaches. They can also cause eye strain. Dark circles have a devastating effect on the appearance. Aloe vera gels are rich in minerals and vitamins that aid in restoring your youthful appearance.

If you're worried about dark circles, you should try aloe vera. It can work in a remarkable method to assist you in getting rid of the under eye dark circles.

Apply pure or in a mix with aloe vera gel and other fruits for dark circles. Check out the surprising results.

ANTI-AGING:

Aloe vera can also be used to combat aging. It's rich in vitamin C as well as vitamin E that helps moisturize the skin and increase its elasticity and firmness. It also reduces wrinkles appearing on the skin, and can make you appear younger and attractive.

Start making use of aloe vera now. The method for using it is exactly identical. Apply aloe vera gel and wash it off after 15 minutes.

Removes stretch marks:

Aloe vera helps to diminish the stretch marks that come with pregnancy. The experts suggest applying aloe vera gels at the point you first notice stretch marks. The marks are an outcome of inflammation. Because it is anti-inflammatory it helps reduce the appearance in stretch marks.

If you're looking for solutions to stretch marks, here's an easy solution to the problem. Apply aloe Vera gel on the skin affected and gently massage it over the affected area. To get the best results, apply it frequently.

3-Hair Care:

Hair is a significant part in expressing our character. So taking care of our hair is equally important. I'll repeat the aloe vera can help to fight hair-related problems.

Prevent hair loss:

Aloe vera is proven to be effective in reducing hair loss. It is a source of enzymes and nutrients that promote growth of hair. These enzymes work to eliminate hair cells that are dead. This helps to promote hair's growth and also helps to preserve moisture.

If you're concerned about your appearance and are worried about the loss of your hair then now is the perfect moment to let go of worrying about it. I've given you the easy and simple solution so take it on. Aloe vera is best utilized in the form of gel. Apply it on the scalp and massage it for about a few minutes. It is not necessary to apply it every day. Make use of it only once the week to benefit.

Treats dandruff:

Aloe Vera can be used to treat the dandruff. Dandruff is a fungal condition of the scalp, which can cause dryness. Aloe vera has anti-fungal and hydrating properties.

Aloe vera can help moisturize your scalp and eliminate dryness. Anti-fungal properties treat dandruff. This is why aloe vera provides an icy effect on your scalp.

Take fresh aloe vera gel. Massage it into your scalp. After 15 minutes wash it off. Because the aloe gel is not oily, so post shampooing with aloe vera are not needed.

Therefore, you should begin using aloe Vera as a home treatment for dandruff.

Treatment for scalp itches:

Aloe vera is also utilized to treat itchy scalp. It helps to keep the moisture in scalp by utilizing its nutrients. Aloe vera helps to remove dead skin cells by its enzymatic activity.

This helps reduce dryness and itching on the scalp. Aloe vera can provide a soothing sensation to your scalp.

Aloe vera can be used as a hair conditioner:

Aloe Vera is an excellent conditioner that can help bring back the shine and natural luster of hair. The mechanism behind its operation is similar to that of. It moisturizes and replenishes the hair, without rendering them oily.

Aloe vera is the main ingredient in the majority of conditioners on the market. However, this homemade conditioner will provide a remarkable service for you. Make use of aloe vera gel in the aftermath of shampooing and let it sit for a several minutes. After that, rinse it out. The result will be healthy silky and smooth hair. You will be able to say, Aloe vera is really an amazing plant.

Aloe vera is a remedy for damaged hair:

Aloe vera gel can also be used to heal damaged hair by the aid of its protein portion. It begins by cleaning the hair of dirt and then the proteins restore hair, making it soft and healthy.

Most people suffer from the problem with damaged hair. Aloe vera provides the most effective remedy. Try it at your home. A gel or juice of aloe vera can help. You'll see the effects after washing it out of your hair.

Aloe vera to treat baldness:

This is specifically targeted at males, Baldness is a prevalent issue for males. Aloe vera has been proven to be beneficial for treating baldness, too. When you are bald, the fall of hair begins at a specific portion of the head and spreads out over.

Aloe vera hydrates the scalp to encourage hair growth and also prevent loss.

4-Dental Care:

Aloe vera can be extremely beneficial in maintaining oral hygiene. It's safe and efficient in preventing and curing oral illnesses. It is beneficial for both inflammations and infections in the mouth cavity.

Gum disease cures:

Aloe vera can be described as a naturally-occurring anti-bacterial. It also has vital nutrients that aid in healing. It can be used for treating mouth ulcers as well as bleeding gums.

If you have bleeding gums, put aloe vera gel and apply it to the fingertip , and gentle massage your gums. Powdered aloe vera may also be mixed with toothpaste. It will make you feel more comfortable after you use it.

For mouthwashes:

The juice of aloe vera can be used to make mouthwash. It eliminates the oral bacteria thanks to the antibacterial and antiviral, and antifungal properties. Vitamin C aids in healing bleeding gums.

It is simple to make at home and does not cause negative side negative effects. It will be delicious with its unique natural taste.

Aloe Vera as an anti-plaque:

The most effective method to prevent gum disease is to stop formation of plaque. Aloe vera is able to decrease the formation of dental plaque. It does this by killing bacteria responsible for plaque.

Dosage and Precautions

Aloe vera is extremely secure for use on the outside. If you're applying it to your skin for cosmetic purposes don't use it daily. It is able to deliver the results you want by using it only once two weeks or max. two times per week, but not more than the recommended amount.

You can apply its clear gel on its own or mixed with other juices of fruit. The aloe vera gel shouldn't exceed one tablespoon for one application.

If you are looking to utilize aloe vera to treat cuts or minor injuries, you can use it every day however, only every other day. If you don't experience noticeable improvement until the third day of treatment, then you should discontinue taking it off. The issue is either very serious or it is not related to the treatment method that is based on Aloe vera.

It could cause allergic reactions on skin however, these reactions are not seen quite often. If you notice irritation or redness on your skin after applying or application of gel aloe vera cleanse it right away. Don't repeat the application.

Chapter 4: Aloe Vera And Kids

Health is a top priority for all. However, we all need to be more mindful of your children's wellbeing. We've previously talked about the therapeutic benefits of aloe vera for adults. It is also utilized to treat ailments of children. The ingredients in Aloe Vera are safe for children of all ages.

Aloe vera can be a bit bitter to the taste. It is very likely that your child will not like it. The fact that they may not like the taste of aloe vera doesn't mean that you can't make use of it for your child. Let me give you how to get it to work. You can add a flavor of your preference to muck up its initial flavor.

Let's look at the health benefits it can bring to children.

Aloe vera and immunity

Aloe vera aids in building immunity by supplying its vitamin. Vitamin C as well as vitamin E can be potent antioxidants which neutralize free radicals that harm health. Aloe vera is also a catalyst for the creation of White blood cells which serve as soldiers for our immune system.

The immune system and digestive system aren't fully developed at the beginning, so they are vulnerable to being affected. Aloe vera is a great way to protect your infant from infection and can help your baby grow stronger.

LAXATIVE:

The children are at the beginning of development. The immune system of children isn't fully matureand therefore they're at chance of contracting a disease.

Aloe vera has been renowned for its ability to laxify over the years. It's also tested with children and found to be to be beneficial. It works exactly the same way for adults. Improves the motility of the gut and softens the stole through the use of its unique composition.

Careful consideration is needed regarding the amount of it. A tiny amount of aloe vera could be a blessing for your children.

Development and growth:

This amazing plant aids in growing and developing children. Aloe vera is a great source of essential nutrients needed in the process of developing.

Two main factors that could hinder normal growth for your children are:

1-DECREASED CELLULAR IMMUNITY

2-LOSS OF A DESIRE

Aloe vera is able to solve both of these issues for us. It aids in protecting against illness and helps promote healthy living. It improves the immune system, making your child stronger and more immune to infections. It can also neutralize free radicals inside the body, which can interfere with normal function of many processes.

A lack of appetite has become a frequent complaint among the children. It could be due to an inability to digest. Aloe vera is a great remedy in this respect. It improves the motility of stomach and aids in the early digestion process, which means that appetite is stimulated.

With the aid of aloe Vera as a supplement, we can look after our children and provide them with all necessary nutrients to develop normally.

Sleep peacefully:

Sleeping peacefully is essential for proper development of children. It is only achievable in the case of a baby who is well-behaved and in good health. Aloe vera is a good source of health for both you as well as your baby.

Aloe vera is a complete health benefit and is good for the entire family.

Treating ALLERGIES in children:

The digestive system and the immune system of a child aren't fully developed in their early years, which means they're at a at risk of developing allergies and infections.

Aloe vera can assist you in this respect. It's equally effective to be used externally by children as it is for adults.

Use a light layer Aloe vera gel on the skin that is affected. It offers an emollient and moisturizing effect for the skin when it is applied externally. It works by killing germs and nourishing the skin with the aid of its nutrients. It aids in healing through the process of synthesizing new cells.

It is safe to use with your kids since the aloe vera plant is safe for kids.

DOSAGE:

Infants and toddlers... 1 ounce per day

3-5 years children...1 teaspoon per day

6-8 years children... 1.5 tea spoons per day

8-12 years children.. 1 tablespoon per day

PRECAUTION:

Children tend to be the most sensitive creatures. It is essential to take care when the use of aloe-vera for kids. These guidelines should be considered when using aloe vera:

1. Aloe vera isn't safe for children younger than 12 months old.

2. A high dose of aloe vera should be prevented.

3. Make sure it is out of the reach of kids.

4. If you do not notice any significant improvement in the regular usage or Aloe vera, you should consult with a physician instead of expanding its use.

5. Do not use aloe vera for persistent issues.

6. Use aloe vera only to treat wounds that are severe.

7. If you notice any type of reaction to the use of it , you should stop using aloe and ask a doctor to get an opinion.

Chapter 5: Veterinary Benefits Of Aloe Vera

The aloe plant is vital for the wellbeing of our four-legged companions. It is utilized in both ways both internally and externally. The mechanism of action is nearly identical to that of humans.

If you have pets , or If you are a lover for animals, then you will certainly enjoy this section.

Aloe vera has many benefits for the internal:

The consumption of aloe vera assists your pet in various ways.

1- Laxative:

Aloe vera is proven beneficial in treating constipation in animals, and also aids in digestion. It also helps combat diarrhea due to its antibacterial properties.

Aloe vera is offered as a juice for pets. For herbivores the aloe vera leaf may be served along with food.

2- Grass sickness:

This is a common disease among horses. It is most common in the summer and spring seasons. The causes are not yet known however there is a different theories that suggest the presence of some kind of toxins in grass can reduce the intestinal motility leading to constipation and poor digestion.

The desire to eat is triggered the feeling of emptiness in the stomach. The gut remains full due to its reduced motility and thus inability to consume more. This condition is known by grass sickness.

In this instance, aloe vera juice is provided in large quantities to improve digestion. This results in a greater appetite and grass sickness being gone.

3. Good for joints and bones:

Arthritis is a condition that causes arthritis of the joints. The joint's protective layer are damaged by aging and becomes inflamed in the future. Aloe vera can help your pet with this condition.

It assists in reducing inflammation, and also helps to promote healing through the creation of new cells near the site of injury.

4- Animal's immunity:

Aloe vera is a must to your pets to boost their immunity since they are more likely to be infected, which is higher than that of human beings. Vitamins in the plant act as antioxidants against free radicals and assist to neutralize their effects.

It also stimulates the production also White blood cells, which fight off bacteria (bacteria virus as well as fungus) and thus cleanses the body.

The gel or leaf of aloe vera is recommended to give your pets every 2 to 3 months in order to strengthen their immunity.

5Aloe vera and diseases:

Animals are extremely prone to contract infections due to their hygiene-related issues and the possibility of transmitting disease are extremely high. Aloe vera is extensively used to fight diseases in animals too. The plant is very suitable for pets since it is virtually non-toxic and has no negative side effects.

6- Infections of the urinary tract:

Animals aren't able to keep their hygiene in check. They are at risk of suffering from Urinary tract infections. Aloe vera is an effective treatment for these kinds of infections.

77 Aloe vera to improve mental and physical health

Aloe vera is extremely refreshing. It improves the physical and mental well-being of your pet. It assists in cleansing their bodies and make them clear of the free radicals. It also aids in digestion, which will result in the delivery of all necessary nutrients to the various organs of the body through blood circulation.

These nutrients are essential to the functioning of the body, so each system functions at its peak and the health is restored.

8. Respiratory infection:

Aloe vera can be used for treating respiratory tract infections. It is also beneficial for persistent illnesses. It kills the agent that causes disease and relieving symptoms by utilizing its vitamins, particularly Vitamin C as well as vitamin E.

External advantages of aloe vera

The long-lasting health benefits of aloe vera are not to be overlooked. The gel of aloe vera is widely applied topically to treat different skin conditions in animals.

1- Anti-parasites:

Aloe vera can be insect repellent that is used for pets. Since animals are usually in unsanitary environments the aloe vera plant helps in keeping mosquitoes out.

Aloe vera is applied to the animal's skin. The animal may not be a fan of the sounds that the spray makes. If that's the scenario, you can apply aloe gel and rub it into the skin and coat of the pet.

2. Care for the fur and skin:

Aloe vera is a great choice for skin care and fur. It softens skin and eliminates the dead cells of skin. It also acts as an conditioner for hair.

All you need to do is apply aloe vera gel on the fur and skin and then massage for a time so that it is absorbed into the skin. Finally, wash it off in a few minutes. After drying , you can be able to feel the softness of fur.

3. To heal cut and sprains:

Animals are susceptible to being injured. Aloe vera, also known as the healer plant is also beneficial in minor injuries and cuts of animals.

Clean the wound using clean tap water. Apply aloe Vera gel to the wound. It will help to disinfect the area of injury and help promote healing through the creation of new cells.

4- Calves hair growth:

The calves can lose hair on their backs. The loss of hair isn't easy to detect. It is usually as patches. Certain veterinarians suggest that this condition could be due to some type of allergic reaction or infection.

Following loss of hair The affected area is exposed to sun's rays and is at chance of sunburn.

In this situation, aloe vera gel is useful. Apply a thin layer of aloe vera gel to the affected area of the skin. It's role is to hold moisture on the skin and stimulate hair growth. Aloe vera gel protects the skin from sunburn. It also treats the root in hair loss.

Animals typically wipe it off however it's okay. It is not a good idea to apply it once more. Certain nutrients are absorbed into the skin, while the remainder enters the digestive tract and aids in treating its primary cause.

5- Itchy dogs:

Certain breeds of dogs are extremely sensitive to bites from fleas. The affected skin is extremely sensitive. of irritation. This type of condition is prevalent in dogs and is only a problem for them.

Aloe vera can be beneficial in this situation. Apply aloe vera gel on the skin that is affected. It provides relief from discomfort and also reduces the allergic reactions. The daily use of the product will result in an improvement.

Dosage recommended:

Rabbit .... 2-4 ml per day

Cat and dog ....10-15 ml per day

Cow and buffalo .... 100-150 ml per day

Horse .... 100-150 ml per day

Goat, sheep, and pig .... 50-70 ml per day

Beware of the following when making use of Aloe vera Animals:

1. Aloe vera is beneficial for everyone, but caution should be exercised when making use of it.

2. Always remember the dose recommended for your pet.

3. Do not give too much to your animal because it can be harmful to health.

4. If Aloe is not working to cure, consult a doctor for advice.

5. Always seek medical advice in the event of injuries that are severe.

6. Always consult your physician prior to using this medication in conjunction with other medicines.

7. Do not use Aloe vera in milk-producing animals, since certain ingredients could appear in blood of the animal.

Chapter 6: How Do I Rely On Aloe Vera?

After you have read the previous chapters I am almost certain that you've decided to make use of aloe vera. You are probably contemplating how to make use of it. In this article, I will give you a variety of recipes for aloe vera. Then you'll be able to appreciate the benefits of this plant.

Aloe vera isn't very good in flavor. It is a good fruit to consume on its own or mixed with other fruits to create the best flavor. It's your choice.

Aloe vera recipe for internal use

It is possible to eat or drink aloe vera in a range of varieties. Here are a few recipes for aloe vera can be made at your home.

Aloe vera juices:

1-Banana strawberry aloe vera Smoothie

It is refreshing for anyone. It's delicious in taste and is healthy for everyone. If you aren't a fan of the taste of aloe Vera and you still want to make use of it, this recipe is perfect for you. Try it out for yourself. I am sure you'll love it.

This recipe is intended for a single serving.

INGREDIENTS:

Milk .... 1 1/2 cup

Banana.......................................1 in number

Strawberries.............................4 in number

Aloe vera..................................2 table spoons

Sugar...According to your taste

Ice .... Half cup

DIRECTIONS:

1. Add all the ingredients to the blender.

2. Blend it for an hour or so until it becomes smooth.

3. Drink immediately and serve.

2 Aloe Vera, orange Juice and

Here's a recipe that is perfect for those who love aloe vera. It's simple, but refreshing and healthy. Try this at your home. I hope that you like it.

INGREDIENTS:

Fresh Aloe vera gel............................. 1-2 table spoon

Fresh orange juice................................ 250 ml

Ice...2-3 cubes

Sugar.. If needed, as per your preference

Lemon..1 in number and medium in size

DIRECTIONS:

1. Take freshly-cut Aloe Vera gels from their leaves.

2. Blend all the ingredients in the blender.

3. Mix it up for 1 minute.

4. Drink immediately and serve.

You could also mix other juices from other fruits to replace orange juice, based on the juice you prefer.

3-Aloe Vera Mango and Coconut smoothie

This is a refreshing summer drink and tastes amazing. If you like mangoes, give it a try. It's extremely cooling and refreshing during the summer. I hope that you like it.

INGREDIENTS:

Coconut milk....................................200 ml

Aloe vera leaf................................... 1 in number and medium in size

Mango chunks................................. Half cup

Honey... 1 Tablespoon

Ice... Half cup

Sugar.. According to your taste

DIRECTIONS:

1. Place all the ingredients into the blender.

2. Mix it well for about 1-2 minutes until it becomes smooth.

3. Drink immediately and serve.

4Aloe vera and honey

Honey when combined with water creates an icy effect. It is also possible to make aloe vera and honey drink. It's simple and simple to prepare, but particular to improve your health. I hope you enjoy this recipe.

INGREDIENTS:

Aloe vera leaf.........................1 in number and medium in size

Honey.....................................50ml

Water.....................................200 ml

Ice .... Half cup

Sugar...................................... If needed, as per your preferences

DIRECTIONS:

1. Blend all the ingredients in the blender.

2. Blend it in 2 mins to get it more smooth.

3. Drink immediately and serve.

It is also possible to experiment with a different fruit of your choice. Be aware of one thing: limit your intake to 2 Tablespoons per day. A high intake of medical plants is harmful.

Mint salad and aloe vera:

Aloe vera is beneficial for health, regardless of the mode of intake. It can be consumed in any style that you like. If you are a regular eater of salad alongside food, you can consider making the form of a salad.

INGREDIENTS:

Fresh Aloe vera gel........................ Extracted from 1 medium sized leaf

Tomato... 1 in number and medium in size

Cucumber.....................................1 in number and medium in size

Mint leaves .... 8-10 in numbers

DIRECTIONS:

Cut the vegetables into pieces and later mix them.

Aloe vera is a plant that has recipes to use externally

Aloe vera is also beneficial for use on the outside. It is a great ingredient to use in many different combinations.

1-Aloe lemon juice and vera mask:

Aloe vera is a regenerative ingredient that also improves the complexion. It also assists in removing those dead cells and makes the skin shiny and smooth. Lemon is a great source of vitamin C as well as having bleaching properties.

This is a rejuvenating and whitening mask. It's incredible for everyone's skin. Its effects are evident shortly after using it.

INGREDIENTS:

Aloe vera leaves................... 2 in total and medium in size

Lemon................................1 in number and medium in size

DIRECTIONS:

1. Extract Aloe vera gel from its leaves.

2. Extract juice from lemons using an extractor.

3. Blend it up to create a smooth mix.

4. Apply it to your face and massage it for an extended period of time.

5. Rinse your face using fresh water within 15 minutes after application.

2-Aloe vera face mask for normal and dry skin:

The mask is also employed to revitalize skin. Honey is also loaded with vital nutrients. Both of these natural ingredients perform admirably when used in combination. Make sure to try it at your own home. It's awe-inspiring. I'll show you how to create it.

INGREDIENTS:

Aloe vera leaf..........................2 in number

Honey...................................... 2 Table spoons

DIRECTIONS:

1. Get fresh gels of aloe vera out of its leaf.

2. Blend aloe vera gel as well as honey together.

3. Apply this mix on the face and the neck the neck area.

4. Keep it for 10 to 15 minutes.

5. Rinse it off using tap water.

3- Aloe vera face mask for normal and oily skin:

This mask is great for those with oily skin. If you suffer from oily skin, my advice to you is to not neglect to apply this mask. After you have used it, you will are in agreement with me. Let me tell you how to create it.

INGREDIENTS:

Aloe vera gel.....................................1 table spoon

Clay...1 table spoon

Tea tree oil..1 drop

Lavender oil......................................1 drop

Fresh water..................................... Half cup

DIRECTIONS:

1. Blend all ingredients together in the bowl.

2. Add water drops as needed, and mix to create an emulsified paste.

3. Apply this paste on the cleansed skin.

4. Allow it to sit for 10 minutes before washing it off with tap water.

4Aloe vera and yogurt:

This yogurt and aloe vera mask is specifically designed to treat sunburns and allergies. It provides a gentle treatment to damaged skin. It is possible to try it at home and reap the advantages.

INGREDIENTS:

Aloe vera leaf..............................2 in number

Chilled yogurt.............................3 table spoon

DIRECTIONS:

1. Extract aloe Vera gel out of its leaves.

2. Mix the aloe vera juice and yogurt in a blender until you have an even mixture.

3. Apply the mixture on the skin affected.

4- Let it sit in place for about 15 mins.

5. Wash it away and notice the improvement.

5- Moisturizing mask:

This mask is a mixture of egg yolk, milk cream as well as aloe Vera juice. The ingredients listed are high in protein and can help moisturize the skin.

It is a great product to use to clean your skin. You'll be amazed at the results.

INGREDIENTS:

Aloe vera gel .... 1 Tablespoon

Milk cream...1 table spoon

Egg yolk...1 table spoon

DIRECTIONS:

1. Mix all ingredients together in the bowel until you achieve an homogenous mix.

2. Apply this on the face and neck.

3. You can leave it for about 15 minutes.

4. Clean it up with tap water.

6- Aloe vera and cucumber eye gel:

This gel is comprised from Aloe vera as well as cucumber. Both of these ingredients are extremely moisturized and are rich in vitamins and are therefore crucial to treat dark under-eye circles.

INGREDIENTS:

Fresh Aloe vera gel .... 1 table spoon

Cucumber .... 1/4 of a medium sized cucumber

DIRECTIONS:

1. Cut cucumber into pieces and put it the blender.

2. Blend it for 1-2 mins until it's smooth.

3. The juice should be filtered out.

4. Then mix 1 table spoon Aloe vera gel in cucumber juice.

5. Make sure to apply it as soon as possible for the best outcomes.

6. If you don't want to use it, keep it refrigerated. It's not safe to store for longer than a day or two.

7. CONTRAINDICATIONS SIDE EFFECTS, AND A DRUG INTERACTION WITH ALOE VERA

The sole focus on the advantages of aloe vera is extremely unfair. It is important to understand the complete benefits of aloe vera before beginning making use of it. Aloe vera is extremely beneficial for health, however it is less prone to adverse effects and is not recommended under certain situations.

For your greater understanding, I'm going to inform you of potential side effects and contraindications of aloe vera.

Contraindications to aloe vera

The use of aloe vera is prohibited in the following circumstances:

1-ALLERGIES:

Beware of using aloe vera when you have an allergy to its constituents. The experts advise against using it even if you are allergic to onions or garlic, as they all belong to the same family.

The long-term use of aloe vera can result in an allergic reaction to the skin. Always make sure to use it with caution. If you suffer from Allergic reactions, the first thing to do is to stop using aloe vera and consult a dermatologist as soon as you can.

2- Pregnancy:

It is recommended not to take aloe vera supplements during pregnancy since it is not safe during the pregnancy. It can cause problems such as:

Aloe vera can lower blood sugar levels that could cause harm to the health of both mother and baby. It is therefore advised not to take Aloe vera during pregnancy.

* Aloe Vera is a laxative agent that can deplete electrolytes, which are essential for both the mother and the baby.

* Aloe vera can cause an uterine contraction, which could be harmful for babies.

Due to the above-mentioned adverse effects, it is recommended not to use aloe vera in your the course of pregnancy. External application has no negative impact on the pregnancy. It doesn't enter the blood circulation when applied topically, and is therefore considered safe.

3- Beast-feeding:

Experts advise to avoid using aloe vera while breastfeeding. You might be wondering what is the reason? The answer for this query is unknown. Studies are ongoing. The presence of any active components in milk has not been yet reported.

To ensure that you are safe It is recommended not to take aloe vera internally while breastfeeding.

4Abdominal cramps

It is not recommended to apply aloe vera to abdominal cramps. Aloe vera helps boost gut motility and aids to treat constipation, and a little discomfort can be felt. In the event of stomach cramps, the aloe can cause the problem to become more serious.

Therefore, avoid using aloe Vera to treat abdominal cramps. Also, consult your doctor to find out the cause and the best way to get rid of it.

5- Intestinal disorders:

Aloe vera and its counterparts may cause irritation to the intestine which is why it's not recommended in patients with intestinal obstruction (usually occurs in older patients) ulcerative colitis, appendicitis.

6- before surgery:

If you are taking aloe vera and you have plans for surgery, you should stop using aloe prior to the surgery. Aloe vera acts as an effective blood thinner that can help prevent blood clotting.

Don't use aloe vera if planning to undergo an operation in the next couple of days, since it can cause bleeding.

Aloe vera has side effects:

Aloe vera offers numerous health benefits, but it is also true the fact that it can cause negative consequences. The use of it externally is nearly completely safe, but its internal use can cause problems. There are a few possible side effects associated with aloe vera

1- Hypoglycemia:

Aloe vera reduces blood sugar levels as it metabolizes glucose in the blood. This is beneficial for people with diabetes since it aids in controlling blood sugar levels. However, excessive consumption of aloe vera can cause hypoglycemia.

Therefore, care must be taken when taking internal aloe vera.

2. Risk of bleeding:

Aloe vera is an anticoagulant in nature. It reduces the formation of platelets that could cause excessive bleeding. Platelets are blood cells that stop bleeding at the point of injury.

In the case of certain diseases, the number of platelets decreases more than usual and the situation arises, we begin making use of aloe vera in a way that is not intended it could cause death.

Therefore, it is essential to be fully informed about the plant prior to making use of it.

3- Dehydration:

Aloe vera helps with constipation by promoting bowel movements. In this case, less of water is taken up by the gut's walls. The long-term use of aloe vera can cause dehydration . It can also lead to a deficiency in vital nutrients.

Long-term and excessive usage of aloe vera is to be kept away from.

4 Allergic reactions:

The long-term use of aloe vera can cause itching and redness to the skin. In this instance, you should stop taking Aloe Vera. Consult a a dermatologist for a proper guidance.

5 - Aloe Vera and liver damage:

The liver is the most important organ of our body. It plays a number of essential roles to ensure the proper functioning of our body. It is able to synthesize protein and other kinds of enzymes. In addition it regulates hormones and aids in the elimination of the toxins. Bile juice, made by the liver assists in the digestion process of food.

Aloe vera was identified as to be hepatotoxic as of 2005. The mechanism behind its action is not yet known. The toxicity caused by Aloe Vera is not serious. It is a self-limiting condition.

Possible drug interactions:

Aloe can work in conjunction with other drugs, so if seeking treatment for any kind of illness, before you use aloe vera you should consult your doctor regarding it. Use it only when it is deemed as safe.

1. Medicines that control sugar:

The condition of diabetes is hyperglycemic. The treatment with drugs help to reduce blood sugar levels, thereby promoting healthy living. Aloe vera is also able to lower blood sugar levels through reducing the glucose-insulin resistance.

If we take aloe vera in conjunction with medication to control sugar levels the combination effect of both can cause hypoglycemia.

Therefore, before you use it, make sure you consult with your doctor . Use only after being approved as safe by your medical professional.

2- Blood pressure-controlling medication:

Diuretics are a specific kind of blood pressure-controlling medications. They help regulate blood pressure. It could cause a drop in potassium levels in the body that is necessary to perform various bodily functions.

Aloe vera can also lower potassium levels to a certain extent when it is used regularly. If aloe vera is combined in conjunction with diuretics, it could be a problem.

Do not forget to inquire with your physician whether you can use aloe vera with blood pressure-lowering medications.

Chapter 7: Aloe Vera Benefits For Childs

When the initial development takes place, each part of the current situation of a child develops into a specific part. We now know that specific supplements play an important role in the growth of a child's cerebrum, body, or even personality, and these supplements can aid or hinder normal development. Surprisingly, the growth of aloe vera does not only help the body's handling and utilization of the primary nutrients needed for health and health, but it can also help in the development of optimal functioning of the many body's cycles , and safeguard the health of your child!

From conception to birth

Prior to the time of origination, organic elements that play significant roles in the proper growth of an embryo and then, following the hatchling's development can create huge differences due to the mental, physical and energetic growth of a child. Before birth, all the nutrients required for the development of nerves, cells and organs must be in place to ensure a proper turn of events and functioning of the framework. If you have adequate supplies of macronutrients and micronutrients during the uterus, the health of a child is able to be enhanced prior to birth, but as a result of improvements after the birth.

Aloe vera's ability to enhance the absorption of supplements and enhance the function of the body's systems to enhance the use of these supplements, it's no surprise that aloe is being studied and studied to determine whether it is safe and effective including aloe vera in the pre-birth program. Similar to every new procedure that takes place in pregnancy, it is important be sure to consult with their physician before introducing aloe vera

to your day-to-day to your daily routine.

The virus known as chickenpox is recognized throughout all over the world and is seen most often in children between the ages of five and 10 years old. As the virus continues to run its course and is cured in a natural way, the application of aloe Vera on the skin can ease discomfort and reduce inflammation that is that is caused by irritation of the skin caused by the virus.

Vitamins

The nutrients required by the developing embryo are extensive. From A to E, each of the nutrients is needed to ensure that the embryo is in the right sequence of events. If there is a deficiency in just one of the nutrients, the consequences could be disastrous. Spina bifida is a physical disorder that may result due to a lack of intake and use of B vitamins. Incorrect growth and the enclosure of the spine causes physical issues that plague the baby with pain and suffering for the rest of his all of. In order to ensure that the child is getting all of the nutrients essential to life by the mother's frenzied eating routine and supplementation, the child will thrive throughout the first year of pregnancy and even into later life.

It is estimated that the World Health Organization estimates that around 250 million preschool children are deficient in vitamin A. In the absence of proper nutrition this

Deficiency could have disastrous effects; each year, 250,000 to 500,000 children lose their eyesight due to Vitamin A deficiencies.

B VITAMINS

B nutrients play an important role in the growth of synapses', nerves and connections, as well as helping to maintain the development of the spine. The bones, blood brain, and the body's natural framework all begin with B-nutrients in the uterus. They are responsible for the development of vision as well as chemical production, as well as the development of teeth in the future All B vitamins are present in abundance throughout the pregnancy.

Vitamins A, C AND E

With the three nutrients C, A C and E having synergistic components that aid one another in promoting the child's healthy course of events and the bones, nerves and blood benefit from the adequate intake of these essential nutrients. Additionally, they help to improve the health of a baby throughout the pregnancy, and even after of these nutrients also help to build solid, secure structures, as well as protecting the baby from illnesses and sicknesses which can hinder the growth and development in the uterus.

Minerals

The essential minerals needed throughout pregnancy don't just ensure mom's physique remains well-nourished and able to deliver and carry a healthy child, but they also provide the assistance needed to improve the baby. From conception to birth ample minerals are needed to ensure that the infant can take care of supplements and produce properly.

Calcium

A lot of people are adamant about calcium in creating and maintaining

to build solid bones. this mineral can be a huge help to other than

bone advancement in utero. Responsible for the growth and arrangement of

the teeth and the skeletal framework an adequate supply of calcium is also required.

necessary for the development of nerves and to aid of their work, just as

the strength of blood's strength. Without calcium-rich supplies the blood's strength is diminished.

Placentas don't offer the hatchling the necessary nutrients to

growth, and may even trigger the growth of blood development, and even lead to the improvement of blood clots.

Iron

The growth of a child's hemoglobin begins in the uterus, and iron plays an important role in the course of things. While it is not a guarantee that the blood is stocked with important components, but iron also helps reduce the risk of illness and reduce the risk in the event of a low birthweight or an untimely birth.

Protein is a vital nutrition for every child, and helps to aid in the proper development and growth of all parts of our brains to system of the body. Children aged between 1 and 8 require an average amount of between 13-19g of protein a day as adolescents and children between nine and eighteen require 34 and 52 grams daily.

Zinc

A vital cerebrum necessity zinc is accountable to enhance the development and growth of the mind as well as every of its parts. Insuring that there is a proper connection between each component of the cerebrum. Zinc helps in the proper sequence of events as well as the working of cells, nerves and pathways

accountable for control of engines for engine control, speech improvement, and cognizance. Additionally, it is required for the production and management of insulin as well as essential enzymatic activities Zinc is a vital mineral required throughout each stage of development.

How Aloe Can Help?

In the course of pregnancy, all the needs and requirements of an enthusiastic mother and her infant's toes and feet. With adequate supplies of each mineral and nutrient being provided through supplementation and diet both mother and baby can be able to develop in the way they want without problem. Aloe will not only aid in to get the necessary minerals and nutrients required for pregnancy by providing supplements of each vital one and can also aid by helping to improve the framework for improvement and working that delivers the supplements and makes use of them as well as increasing the availability of the nutritional supplements consumed. The extraordinary phytochemicals in aloe allow the mother-to-be and baby to benefit from a greater intake of minerals and nutrients which makes them less likely to suffering from deficiencies throughout the pregnancy process and after birth. In addition to the benefits of the experience of pregnancy using aloe hasn't just been shown to decrease the likelihood of nausea, but also helps in maintaining a healthy electrolyte levels in both the mother and the child and reduce the risk of drying out that may be caused by morning sickness.

Disease and Disease Prevention

Children are exposed to a variety of microbes, organisms, and infections that may cause illness and ailments. With vulnerable frameworks that are less well-developed and effective than those of adults, children are likely to be susceptible to illness by being open to spots, individuals and other things that not have much influence on resilient frameworks. In addition to the issue of immunity Children are typically exposed to each other in closed spaces like classrooms when they are playing The germs found in air or on the surface are easily transferred between children and are able to spread throughout an entire group even when there is no sign of symptoms. To fight the withdrawal of disease it is important to focus on

On vulnerability is an absolute requirement for every child, from right from birth until adolescence.

Immunity

Vitamin C has for a long time been recognized as a strong insusceptibility that can aid the body's ability to anticipate and treat ailments. Because this nutrient plays significant roles in the construction of the body's defenses as well, it is by distant possibility the primary nutrients that work to strengthen the body's insusceptible structure. The complete spectrum of minerals and nutrients in addition to adequate amounts of sugars, proteins and fats, are essential to support the body's normal functioning, and when an insufficiency occurs, resulting in an imbalance or impairment of structure functioning and protecting the body, it are also weakened. By consuming a balanced diet and supplements, that the body is able to get what it needs to function effectively and efficiently, the body's defense system can be restored to its normal state but also make use of specific supplements that function as amazing protections to enhance the body's protections more.

Children require vitamin C to ensure optimal growth and development as well as for the maintaining a healthy immune system that is able to fight against disease and illness. The recommended daily dose to take vitamin C in children ranges in the range of 15-25 mg kids ranging from one to eightyears old, and 45-75 mg in the case of children and adolescents aged 9-18 years old.

With aloe vera's innovative mix of specific phytochemicals, the aid it provides to the vulnerable framework goes well beyond the results you get from basic nutritional advice. These powerful cancer prevention drugs help to prevent contamination, but it also assists the body keep up with solid and perfect blood. They also protect against negative changes that can occur at the level of cells. Assisting the body's ability to pinpoint the needs of the body's framework and organs Aloe vera can combat disease while improving health.

Bacterial Infections

Exposure to microscopic creatures is a common occurrence. As a child's day-to- everyday life, this vulnerability can cause havoc on an overpowered and insusceptible framework. With a fragile, juvenile-invulnerable framework which is focused on removing the multitude of microorganisms which are inhaled and retained throughout the day, children are extremely susceptible to the spread of infections caused by bacteria.

If the illness takes hold on the skin, air routes, blood, or skin bacteria, they can develop into colds, pussy wounds, or real sicknesses. While a healthy lifestyle and washing hands during the course of the day may reduce the risk of contracting bacterial infections Aloe may assist in decreasing the risk considerably.

With the help of inCredible phytochemicals which act around as antibacterial experts and cleanses your blood from microorganisms and reduce the risk of opening to microbes throughout the body. In battling off the contamination caused by openness to bacteria both inside and outside, aloe has been proven to be effective in the removal of the blood, skin and the surprising respiratory structure of harmful microbes that could develop into real illnesses. Assisting the cancer prevention substances of the vitamins A, C and E, which are absorbed through aloe vera, this easy increase in the vulnerability procedure can effectively safeguard the health of your body's cells and structures as well as preventing the spread of infections.

Infections Viral

Influenza and viruses can be dangerous and insufferable for adults but in children the infection can be deadly. Because there aren't any restorative medications available to fight infections viruses, they must be treated by anticipating. Invulnerability to infection is vital to reduce the chance of getting an infection and a strong resistance could lower the severity and length of a viral illness too. A diet that is comprised of healthy foods

soil products which are rich in essential susceptibility-supporting supplements A resistant framework will perform as planned and to protect against infections as well as their contaminants. The minerals A, C and E, as well as the minerals zinc and iron can aid in preventing infections by assisting in the development of a safe framework and ensuring that the essential supplements needed for insurance are readily available.

The absorption of these vital anti-viral minerals and nutrients can be improved through the use in the use of Aloe Vera.

Aloe vera is also able to increase the immunity to diseases by providing antiviral specialists who can help treat viral infections inside the body. No matter if the infection is visible on the skin or attempting to take hold of the inside aloe vera's phytochemicals that fight viruses help in eliminating the infectious infection, but also aid in enhancing the body's defenses. Both on the inside and outside the body, aloe's antiviral experts help to prevent the infection from spreading and aloe's array of immune-suppression supplements can further aid the immune system and improve its effectiveness.

This combination of protection and security reduces the risk of viruses that could be a threat to every organ or framework, protecting children from an infection and also decreasing the severity of an illness that may have been effectively treated. The recommendation for children's use of aloe vera varies but generally, it is believed to be safe in the amount of half-a-tsp daily. This amount could be incrementally increased as the child progresses into youth. The daily portion of a child of aloe can provide the necessary protection against insusceptibility and phytochemicals that aid the body to fight infections. This portion could be increased when the child is suffering from an illness and its manifestations. The daily portion consumed by teens regularly can be increased in the time of illness, before returning back to the same daily portion after the illness has passed.

Serious Disease

Children aren't protected from the real illnesses that affect adults. In the absence of a strong, resistant framework and cells in the body's body can transform from healthy to unhealthy. The upgrading of the vulnerable framework and safeguarding that the body is safe from these harmful changes is crucial to protect children's health and progress. With antibacterial and antiviral experts who demonstrate their ability to protect against illness and assist in establishing a healthy structure and aloe

vera does not only provide support for the specific frameworks that protect health, but it also reduces the risk of cell changes level. Fantastic cancer prevention drugs that protect against contamination could aid in maintaining cell health and reduce the frequency of cell-related changes which trigger illness and illness. It is a rich source of minerals and nutrients which are expected to aid in this Aloe vera also provides the cancer-prevention agents believed to improve cell health and the functioning of the framework, helping with the prevention of genuine illness and diseases.

Proper Growth and Development

Children require proper nutrition to ensure the proper growth and development of all things in the cerebrum as well as unresolved questions regarding chemical and framework. Because the body is comprised of synergistic structures that depend on one another for support any insufficiency in one supplement could trigger an impact that is felt in a variety of areas of development.

The most frequent deficiencies observed in children are those related with vitamin D and B vitamins and iron. However, the signs and symptoms caused by nutritional deficiencies are quite similar to common illnesses that children and their parents. ADHD as well as poor speaking development, fatigue diminished cognition, chronic illnesses and so on. All of these can be traced to serious nutritional deficiencies in vitamins and minerals.

Aloe vera may assist in ensuring the proper growth and development of a child in various ways. With an abundance of basic supplements and the benefit that it has a higher retention rate than other supplements as well, aloe vera can be capable of assisting by ensuring that the body's structures are functioning well and remain free of difficult medical issues that could lead to formative maladies.

Hormones and Growth

The pituitary organ has responsibility for the creation of chemical substances and their emission throughout the body. If this chemical is not functioning properly, it could cause a slow digestion, a slow development related to insulin, as well as delayed puberty. Naturally, the nutritional demands for the proper functioning of the pituitary gland are frequently ignored in the normal American eating habits. Nutrient E, along with the minerals manganese and magnesium aid in ensuring the proper functioning of the pituitary organ and also the creation of substances that are essential for proper development. These nutrients are often present in mixed greens as well as whole leafy vegetables and are burnt-through in sufficient amounts through the proper eating habits. Aloe vera is not only a guarantee that these vital supplements are available, but it also aids in the production and diffusion of those chemical compounds through the cardiovascular framework and the nerve communication that transfer the signs of the pituitary organ as well as the body. Through the specialized working of the neuronal cells that result from the phytochemicals present by aloe and vera, cerebrum as well as every body's structure can transmit information better; this results in a further development of chemical formation and guideline mental working and mental clarity.

Cognitive Development

With various elements that consolidate to give kids everything identified with thought, feeling, and mind-set, the cerebrum is one space of wellbeing that should come first for development and advancement. The mind goes about as a control community that can coordinate a kid's improvement actually, however mentally and genuinely too. With aloe vera's arrangements of B nutrients, and the extra amino acids and supplements that further develop B-nutrient ingestion, various mind exercises improve, including the guideline and improvement of feelings and mood.

Mood and Depression

While there are various assessments that propose that drug medicines can assist with further developing episodes of misery, tension, consideration problems, etc, it can assist with understanding that plentiful supplies of the supplements that help cerebrum wellbeing can streamline the working of the cycles constrained by the cerebrum and then again, inadequacies of those fundamental supplements can bring about breaking down. One of the primary gatherings of supplements that have been related with bliss and sorrow are those of the B assortment. Because

 the B nutrients assume significant parts in the advancement of "feel better" chemicals like serotonin and dopamine, and furthermore add to the appropriate turn of events and working of the nerve cells in the mind, how much B nutrients burned-through in the eating regimen can affect the solidness of mind-set and assist with mitigating episodes of depression.

Aloe vera gives B nutrients and fundamental supplements that join to help cerebrum wellbeing, sensory system working, and correspondence inside the mind and between the mind and body. Aloe vera has been displayed to further develop sadness, lessen nervousness, work on intellectual working, and limit pressure among youngsters. The fundamental supplements that are given by aloe vera additionally assist with working on cardiovascular wellbeing and blood quality, which can add to better framework working and limit the danger of raised circulatory strain, frequently connected with raised tension levels, disturbances in manners of thinking, and higher occurrences of stress. The suggested every day portion of 1/2–1 tablespoon of aloe vera can give a kid benefits identifying with state of mind and enthusiastic prosperity. Youngsters can devour a steadily expanded day by day portion between 1–2 tablespoons of aloe vera for further developed state of mind benefits.

Skeletal and Muscle Development

The critical stores and supplies of fundamental supplements are basic for the legitimate development of the skeleton and solid frameworks of each developing kid. Minerals like calcium, iron, magnesium, manganese, and a lot more are used by the body to give the system and backing in the advancement of bones and tissues, while various nutrients and fundamental supplements further advance the appropriate working of this formative interaction. The strong framework likewise relies upon the dietary admission of nutrients, minerals, and macronutrients to grow appropriately, assisting with shaping and keep up with the bulk that offers the help for the skeletal framework. These two frameworks cooperate to offer the help a developing body needs to sit, stand, move, and play. With lacks of significant supplements, however, these two frameworks endure and unleash devastation on the body and life of a creating youngster; in the midst of hardship, the stores of calcium get exhausted from bones and the body can go to existing bulk when needing protein and amino acids. Assisting with working on the body's capacity to ingest and

keep up with appropriate stores of fundamental bone-and muscle-building supplements, a sound eating regimen wealthy in entire food varieties that give fundamental micronutrients and macronutrients required for bone and muscle wellbeing can be made more productive through the basic expansion of aloe. The suggested every day portion of 1⁄2–1 tablespoon of aloe vera can furnish a youngster with nutritive advantages, improving development and improvement, and adolescents can burn-through a progressively expanded day by day portion between 1–2 tablespoons of aloe vera.

Nutrition

Without an uncertainty, sustenance assumes a significant part in the general working of the body. Without satisfactory supplies of the body's necessary supplements, inadequacies and dysfunctions result. For kids, the impacts are undeniably more genuine on the grounds that the lacks and disturbs in the eating routine reason issues in youth, yet can spell fiasco for a lifetime too. To keep up with ideal wellbeing, an emphasis on nourishment outperforms the body's essential necessities and can assist with forestalling various hazardous medical problems that can unfavorably influence the existence of a creating child.

Many youngsters who consistently devour the standard American eating regimen (precisely alluded to by its abbreviation, SAD) loaded up with sodium, sugar, and refined carbs fight with normal ailments and sickness that debilitate their body's frameworks and cutoff their capacities all through life. From heftiness and diabetes to respiratory complexities and hypersensitivities, the consequences of ailing health can make difficulties that influence nature of life.

Obesity

One out of each three youngsters younger than eighteen is presently viewed as overweight or stout. With these stunning insights, pediatricians are diverting their concentration from proposals that essentially urged more exercise to an accentuation on better nourishment. Without legitimate sustenance, a kid does not have the energy and actual capacity to take part in work out, making hindrances that lead to a pattern of less active work and more significant impacts of hunger that further compound weight-related issues.

With the positive consequences of a nutritious eating routine having displayed to work on each space of physical and emotional well-being, the attention on nourishment in kids is one that is well supported.

With a day by day diet that incorporates entire food sources, the body can work appropriately and better control each physical and mental capacity, limiting the dangers related with unhealthiness. Of course, aloe vera's parts have been displayed to additional help a nutritious eating routine, further develop energy levels, and aid every one of the body's frameworks that are engaged with keeping up with legitimate wellbeing and ideal functioning.

Diabetes

Type 1 and type 2 diabetes are insulin-related sicknesses that can prompt genuine confusions and restrictions in the existence of a youngster. Regardless of whether the illness is hereditary (type 1) or created (type 2), a nutritious eating regimen that spotlights on working on the body's capacity to manage insulin and keep up with blood wellbeing is critical. Once alluded to as grown-up beginning diabetes, type 2 diabetes is currently being analyzed in kids at more youthful ages consistently. For instance, there were no youngsters determined to have this sickness in 1980, and an expected 60,000 analyzed in 2012. With this developing issue, the attention on anticipation and treatment of type 2 diabetes is currently being tended to by pediatricians and putting a developing liability on guardians. Handled food varieties loaded with exorbitant sugars are being given to the present kids to each supper and nibble, and the outcome can be cataclysmic in the delicate, creating arrangement of a youngster. A mix of sound sustenance, ordinary exercise, and aloe vera can assist with keeping away from the beginning of diabetes and limit the complexities that emerge thus. While a doctor ought to be counseled before the execution of another regular or therapeutic expansion to a diabetic way of life, the overall proposal for aloe vera utilization would be 1/2–1 tablespoon day by day for youngsters, step by step expanding to a day by day portion of 1–2 tablespoons of aloe vera for teens.

By assisting the body With handling food varieties, keep up with clean blood, and direct how much glucose in the circulation system, aloe vera can help the all body's cycles identified with assimilation, supplement handling, and glucose guideline. These advantages straightforwardly work on the wellbeing and prosperity of a youngster, further developing the exact cycles that are identified with diabetes. With

 added benefits that further develop invulnerability, streamline framework working, and further develop the blood stream, chemical creation, and retention and usage of fundamental supplements, aloe might be one of the best

treatment supports the course of working on the body's capacity to work with diabetes.

High Blood Pressure

Like diabetes and stoutness, hypertension was once considered as a condition that happened distinctly in grown-ups. Anyway this condition is turning out to be an ever increasing number of pervasive in youngsters, striking teenagers and kids as youthful as five. With the developing measurements that give no indication of hypertension being controlled or limited, consideration is currently being centered around the causes and anticipation. Knowing the unsafe impacts of sugar, fats, and added substances in handled food sources on the cardiovascular framework's parts and working, the fault is being put on the weight control plans of these youthful people. Through an eating routine of entire food sources, liberated from synthetics, colors, additives, and added sugars and fats, a youngster can flourish without the worry of hypertension, and aloe can help in each progression of anticipation and treatment.

Rich in nutrients, minerals, and cancer prevention agents, aloe vera isn 't simply ready to assist with lessening the rate of hypertension through adjusting supplement insufficiencies and further developing the cardiovascular framework's working, yet additionally by assisting with keeping up with blood wellbeing in various ways. Fatty substances, glucose levels, and hurtful plaque-storing arrangements found in the blood all join to deliver unsafe results inside the cardiovascular framework, raising the danger of growing high blood pressure.

With aloe vera 's capacity to direct glucose levels, diminish how much awful cholesterol (LDL) while raising great cholesterol levels (HDL), and viably scrub the blood of greasy parts that stop up and confound the cardiovascular framework's working, aloe is one of the most valuable augmentations to a youngster's eating routine. Further working on a kid's capacity to battle hypertension, aloe vera empowers assimilation and utilization of explicit supplements like calcium, zinc, and magnesium that straightforwardly advance the blood's wellbeing just as the nerve framework's and cardiovascular framework's working wherein the blood assumes significant parts. Through an eating routine of supplement thick, normal food sources that contribute fundamental supplements, liberated from handling and added substances, a youngster's blood and body benefit enormously in various ways, one being a lower hazard of hypertension. The suggested day by day portion of 1/2–1 tablespoon of aloe vera can furnish a youngster with pulse benefits, while teenagers might require a slowly expanded day by day portion between 1–2 tablespoons of aloe vera for further developed circulatory strain benefits.

Fatigue

Without an uncertainty, your eating regimen is straightforwardly identified with your energy level. With a quality eating regimen, the supplements the body needs are at any point present, taking into consideration the bones, muscles, and mind to be locked in on request without issue. With a horrible eating routine ailing in fundamental supplements, the outcome can be ongoing weariness that restricts a youngster's capacity and want to take part in actual work. While this might appear as though an inconsequential circumstance that is detached to just specific marks of inadequacy in a kid's life, the outcomes are not really time specific.

When the body is lacking in fundamental supplements, the weakness that outcomes can be felt throughout the span of days, weeks, and even months. Lacking supplies of the supplements required prompts underuse and brokenness of each framework and capacity in the body, and the body's actual sign of these inadequacies and dysfunctions is decreased energy levels. With little energy and less movement coming about, the body can start to encounter decay, further adding to episodes of weakness and idleness, and the cycle proceeds endlessly until the lacks are corrected.

Through its own arrangement of nutrients, minerals, amino acids, and amazing phytochemicals that go about as cancer prevention agents, aloe vera can assist with conveying genuinely necessary supplements. Added to an eating routine of entire food sources that contribute the main part of macronutrients and micronutrients required for a kid to flourish, aloe can further develop energy levels and diminish the occurrence of weakness. Every single framework all through the body can work appropriately through the help of supplements, chemicals, and phytochemicals that aloe gives— regardless of whether the upgrades are a consequence of further developed insusceptibility, abundant supplies of supplements, worked on supplement retention, worked on enzymatic movement, or decreased cancer-causing action inside cells. The advantages to the body's energy levels can be seen through further developed consideration and concentration, higher energy levels, worked on metabolic working, and expanded capacity of the bones and muscles to fill fundamental roles required for action and recovery.

Sleep

Sleep is significant for ideal wellbeing. Without adequate rest, both as far as sum and quality, the psychological and actual wellbeing of a kid can be unfavorably impacted. With brokenness unleashing ruin on everything from processing, state of mind, concentration, conduct, and digestion, a kid experiencing lacking rest can carry on with an existence of strife. With basic changes and the execution of solid propensities, any kid can receive the rewards of tranquil evenings' rest that permit the body and psyche to straighten out, recharge, and revive, assisting any youngster with rediscovering the fun of youth consistently.

Great rest propensities during adolescence can proceed with well all through adulthood as well.

Nutritional Needs and Functions

The sustenance a kid gets from his suppers for the duration of the day can significantly affect the rest cycle. With a daily practice of consistently set dinners and bites that furnish the body with sufficient energy supplies for the duration of the day, the body can tighten its reactions to boosts as a youngster approaches sleep time. With the last supper being given something like one hour before a kid's sleep time, assimilation can happen well before the youngster floats off to rest. The typical movement of assimilation (and any antagonistic responses that could prompt "stomach inconveniences") happen a long time before the body starts to rest and unwind; without the obstruction of stomach related cycles or issues, the body can nod off and stay unconscious, receiving the rewards of the supportive supplements devoured in the last supper of the day.

Physical Activity and Energy Levels

With actual work, the body can utilize its stores of energy, and it relies upon the body's regular rest processes as a period of fixing the body and cerebrum and getting ready energy stores for the next day. With energy used, the body and brain can rest all the more serenely while the"in the background" breakdown and recharging of supplements utilized by the body's organs and frameworks can occur. Through the normal rest patterns of a kid, the degrees of energy are directed, making energy accessible for utilize whenever it is required. Without sufficient rest, the muscles, bones, and mind start to moderate energy, limiting energy levels accessible for energy yield. With sufficient rest, however, the body can flourish, reestablishing an equilibrium of supplements that give the fuel to the functions of the whole body's organs, frameworks, and processes.

Mental Functioning, Mood, and Behavior

Its an obvious fact that the nature of one 's rest can decidedly or contrarily influence conduct and state of mind. With sufficient rest, mind working, discernment, concentration, and conduct improve, and the conduct of all around rested youngsters is straightforwardly reflected in their temperament, school execution, and associations with friends, specialists, and family. This causes circumstances wherein a kid can receive the rewards of positive criticism that add to a pattern of better execution, more sure input, thus on.

Conversely, an absence of rest can deliver inconsistent dispositions, mental weakness, radically weakened concentration and consideration, and may even bring about explosions and social surprises. These manifestations influence a kid's current circumstance, however can likewise make inward tension and confidence issues. Helpless rest propensities can make a negative input cycle, coming about because of helpless conduct and execution, bringing forth regrettable criticism that just further sustains the cycle. Being concentrated on increasingly more consistently, the association among rest and burdensome problems, uneasiness, and consideration issues produce similar outcomes: Sleep is significant for the emotional well-being and ideal working of the creating cerebrum in children.

How Aloe Can Help

Aloe vera can assist with processing, direct glucose levels, and diminish the frequency of stomach related difficulties through its arrangement of phytochemicals, however it can likewise further develop a youth's nature of rest through its amino acids like tryptophan that assist with delivering the rest related chemicals that permit the mind and body to unwind and travel through the

proper phases of rest as planned. With the utilization of aloe vera, not exclusively are the actual stores of fundamental supplements upheld through the one of aloe's very own kind arrangement nutrients, minerals, and phytochemicals, however the advantages to rest all through the sleep time routine can be great as well.

In kids, the most common way of "slowing down" at sleep time can be filled with variances in state of mind, fervor, and energy, prompting a difficult time that is everything except helpful for rest. Aloe vera's quieting amino acids like tryptophan can quiet the body and cerebrum, and its glucose balancing out advantages can assist your youngster with accomplishing rest effectively, securely, and normally. As far as mind-set and conduct in kids, aloe vera can likewise give positive outcomes the help of the psychological cycles and the development of fundamental chemicals that assist youngsters with profiting from better intellectual working, stable temperament, and less burdensome disorders.

Recipes

Great Green Berry Blast

This incredible tasting smoothie is loaded with nutrients, minerals, amino acids, catalysts, and cell reinforcements to improve and secure a kid's by and large health.

Ingredients Serves 4

1⁄4 CUP ALOE VERA JUICE

2 cups natural apple juice

1⁄2 cup cleaved spinach

1⁄2 cup blueberries

1⁄2 medium apple, stripped and cored

Combine all fixings in a blender. Mix until smooth.

Sweet Strawberry Shake

Kids will cherish this supplement rich tidbit, which upholds the working of the whole body's cycles, particularly the brain!

INGREDIENTS SERVES 4

1⁄4 cup aloe vera juice

2 cups unsweetened vanilla almond

milk 1 cup frozen strawberries

2 tablespoons ground flaxseed

Combine all fixings in a blender. Mix until smooth.

Cough-Calming Cooler

You can assist your kid with beating a hack or quiet respiratory brokenness without over-the-counter hack syrups. This normal cure contains anthocyanins and cancer prevention agents that add to the

respiratory framework's working, alongside honey's normally happening antibacterial and antimicrobial properties.

INGREDIENTS

SERVES 2

1/4 cup aloe vera juice

2 CUPS FERMENTED CHAMOMILE TEA, CHILLED

1/2 cup frozen blueberries

1/2 cup frozen blackberries

Chapter 8: How To Grow Aloe Vera?

Once you have a complete understanding of the plant that is a miracle You must be able to decide to utilize it. It is now a matter of where you can get it whether in the marketplace, the garden or further. It's much more effective if it is fresh. Conserved aloe vera is depleted of certain essential nutrients.

My suggestion is to plant it in your own home. It's the only way to have fresh aloe vera any time. It can be planted in your garden. If you don't have a space in your yard In that instance, you can plant it in the doorway, since it thrives when kept within the door. A sufficient amount of sunlight is essential for this plant, so put it where it will be in a position to receive sunlight effectively.

Growing Aloe Vera

Aloe Vera is grown all around the globe because of its incredible advantages. It is easy and accessible for anyone. It's not a problem about it at all. In this chapter , you'll be given a step-by-step guide to grow Aloe Vera from the comfort at home simple and simple. It doesn't require any skills whatsoever. All you need to do is follow the easy steps to create an aloe plant. In the beginning, you'll be required to have the of the following items:

1-A pot that has a drainage hole in the bottom

2. Drain the soil properly

3-Aloe Vera Seed/Small Baby Clone of Aloe Vera/Aloe vera leaf

4-Watering source

Be sure to have all the above listed items with you. Let's begin to plant aloe vera step-by-step. First , take the pot that has a drainage holes in the bottom and then place the soil inside and leave a small amount on top. Dig the soil, then plant the baby aloe vera leaf/seed into the soil. Be aware of one thing: don't give it water for the first couple of hours. After that, water it to the maximum level of the pot, until it starts to drain.

Take care of Aloe Vera

Aloe Vera is a plant that has a high water content, so it is able to freeze easily in cold winter weather. The ideal climate for growing aloe vera is a neutral environment. It can also be grown in hot climates. It requires lots of sunlight for it to flourish. It is better to place it into a container, instead of plant the plant in an unfenced field in order to be capable of placing it inside your doors in the harsh winter conditions.

It doesn't require any fertilizer. However, if you would like to fertilize your soil to improve the development of your garden, provide phosphorus rich fertilizer at least every year, during the spring months.

You don't have to work hard to get it. Make sure not to overwater it. Let the soil dry before watering again. Overwatering is a risk on your garden.

* The yellow leaf is a indication of excessive watering.

* The brown leaf is a indication of a decrease in sun light.

If you notice any of these symptoms, eliminate the root cause as soon as possible to achieve better outcomes.

The leaf is being cut

Begin by cutting the outermost leaves first. Before cutting the leaf, ensure that the leaves are mature and soft.

If your aloe vera tree has grown to a full size and you are eager to use it. It is easy to use using the sharpest knife and cutting the leaf. Let it rest for a second. Aloe vera leaf is not very user-friendly, so you should use rubber gloves to shield your hands. Also, care must be taken when cutting the leaf so as is not to cut the leaf's edge.

Don't be concerned about the injury to your plant. It will heal itself on its own. Even though new leaves don't develop at this point, but the wounds are shut. New leaves begin to grow from the center of the plant. Cutting leaves will interfere with the development of the new leaves.

After removing the aloe vera leaves off the plant, wash it out to get rid of dirt. Don't be afraid by the leaves that are horny. Place the leaf of aloe vera in the cut board, with it upside down . The first step is to remove the sharp edges. Run your knife lengthwise underneath the leaf on the outer layer and cut it off.

Take the Aloe vera gel from the leaves and apply it. It can be preserved with refrigeration, but the best method to absorb all the essential nutrition from this plant is to eat it fresh.

Using Aloe Vera Pulp

Get the pulp of aloe vera from the leaf by squeeze it. Its gel has received all the attention throughout the ages. The gel is able to be applied on the skin to treat therapeutic and cosmetic reasons. It is also used orally for the treatment of various conditions.

You'll be relieved to know it's suitable for children. Another benefit of the aloe plant is that it's great for the health of your pet and pets in the same manner as it is for your family and you.

Chapter 9: Chronic Diseases

Heart disease, stroke abnormal growth and diabetes and stoutness are among the most commonly recognized chronic illnesses across the United States today. With of 117 million Americans today claiming to suffer from one or more of these diseases, more attention is being paid on strategies to combat. With a wide array of remarkable wellness blends, supported by a long track record of success in the treatment and treatment of real ailments Aloe Vera may be able to aid in the ongoing health crisis and improve the health and well-being of millions of people today and for a very long time to in the future.

Heart Disease

The primary cause of deaths across the globe is heart disease that is the most common cause of death, with an average of 17.3 million people dying from coronary disease every year. Researchers across the globe have been battling for years trying to discover the precise reasons behind the diseases that cause coronary disease in general. The entire cardiovascular system is affected by the onset of a cardiovascular disease and six types of coronary disease have been linked to each that affects a different area within the heart.

Coronary heart disease, a condition of blood vessels that supply the heart muscle is the most common of all cardiovascular illnesses.

Cerebrovascular condition is disorder of blood vessels that provide blood to the brain.

Peripheral arterial diseases affect the blood vessels which supply blood to the legs and arms.

Rheumatic fever is caused the streptococcal infection and can cause damage to the heart's muscle and valves.

Congenital heart defects are abnormalities of the heart's structure which are present during the development process before birth.

Deep vein thrombosis refers blood clots within leg veins, which dislodge and then move towards the lungs, heart, or brain, leading to an embolism in the pulmonary tract.

To reduce the number of annual deaths that result from heart disease The World Health Organization has recognized prevention as the most effective method of protection against the risk of developing a cardiovascular disease. About a fifth of heart disease cases result from genetic causes this means that the majority of cases are the result of lifestyle choices. The factors that can contribute to the development of coronary illnesses include inadequate eating pattern as well as smokingcigarettes, and drinking alcohol.

Diet plays an essential role in the progression of heart disease by creating real forerunners of the disease"turn of events. The formation of greasy stores in the vein dividers throughout the body. the food choices and conditions that result due to a long-standing history of poor eating habits have been shown to cause a deterioration in the regions in the heart that are most affected by the disease , by creating these fat deposits and promoting their growth over long period of time.

Even those who do not have a heart problem should pay attention to the physical and nutritional aspects that improve overall health of the heart. With a healthy lifestyle, regularly exercising and a daily intake of aloe vera The heart is the one responsible for the overall health and well-being of the whole body, is able to remain healthy and to function throughout one's existence!

Hypertension, high pulses and high blood lipids obesity, and diabetes are all recognized as factors that contribute to the development of cardiovascular disease. In addition to having a number of negative effects on the general health of a person and general health, these ailments can cause an unintentional disruption in the body's normal balance of sugars, fats and cholesterol. With these three elements of blood having high fixation and the vein dividers containing larger cholesterol (or plaque) stores can hinder the normal development of the circulatory system and increase the risk of developing cardiovascular disease.

Aloe Can Help

With an incredible array of essential supplements and amazing phytochemicals, the aloe vera plant can improve your overall health of the body, improve the body's synergistic structure and eliminate blood, which is a key factor in decreasing the likelihood of suffering from cardiovascular disease. Because weight and diabetes play important roles in the progression of heart disease and heart disease, it is crucial for anyone who is living an approach to life that is beneficial for the conditions to make an honest effort to minimize the elements that contribute to their condition as well as to make the necessary steps to reverse the disease. In both these areas Aloe Vera can assist tremendously.

Most people believe that citrus fruits such as lemons and oranges are the source of the highest amount of vitamin C however, they may be shocked to learn that strawberries have higher levels of vitamin C than oranges , and contain a range of other phytochemicals that are helpful in building immunity and fighting against disease and illness.

Aloe vera provides nutritional supplements that aid the body to keep up with the normal functioning of the framework and, consequently, aiding the obese or diabetic sufferer in reducing the effects of these frameworks. For instance, aloe's vitamins A and C are essential for healthy functioning.

C and E may help in reducing the pressure of oxidative by the ailments while also helping to reduce the risk of. The B vitamins in Aloe and the K nutrients work together to improve overall health and well-being by keeping pace with healthy nerve cells and an the proper connection between neurons and brain.

Obesity is among the most frequent health risks associated with chronic diseases. The condition can not only make it difficult to live a healthy life by restricting things that can otherwise improve overall health, but the burden and energy needed to manage it could create unnecessary stress on organs in the body.

All of these nutrients help to make sound lifestyle decisions through further enhancing energy levels (supporting actions) as well as limiting cravings for unhealthy food sources as well as assisting with the consumption of the essential nutrients and enhancing the body's capacity to flush away fat and build muscles, all of which help to bring the body back to the state of optimal wellbeing. By supplying essential minerals such as iron, calcium as well as magnesium, the aloe protects the body's most important elements like blood, muscle tissues, bone, and tissue. Without the power of these fundamental parts, illness or low energy may cause unfavorable living, such as latency. It is also making the body more susceptible to the onset of a variety of illnesses that may also cause irritation to conditions that contribute to cardiovascular diseases.

The fundamental arrangements of aloe vera that encourage further developed cardiovascular wellbeing are found in the phytochemicals explicit to aloe that go about as cholesterol-improving, blood-purging specialists. Aloe's effects being studied and proven to enhance blood cholesterol levels and fatty substance levels and all the blood lipid levels (all being the most prominent forerunners of cardiovascular disease) it is possible to see the way that aloe can help in strengthening the immune system of a patient in risk and reduce the risk of developing cardiovascular disease.

cardiovascular disease is significant. By taking a regular and consistent day-to-day intake of about 1-3 tablespoons of aloe vera, a good quantity of the minerals, nutrients and cancer-prevention agents and phytochemicals that reduce the chance of advancing of coronary disease is available throughout the body.

Stroke

As with a cardiovascular problem which results from a decreased circulation of oxygen and blood for the heart. Stroke can be described as a"cerebrum attack" which results due to a decrease in the flow of oxygen and blood into the brain. The United States, there is a common one-stroke event, similar to clockwork, and one stroke that triggers death at regular intervals. On average, there are 795,000 strokesper year, with females having 55,000 more of strokes than men each year. Since strokes result from the aftermath of an injury to the cardiovascular structure and are typically combined with those that result from cardiovascular diseases.

If you want to add aloe vera your coffee, water as well as tea or sprinkle it on your favorite salads and side dishes the natural beauty is a great addition to any dish.

integrated into your routine. Tastes similar to water, this flavorless and innocuous addition may go unnoticed however it offers a lot of benefits to all areas of your day-to-day life!

Different kinds of Strokes

Strokes are classified into two categories (ischemic or hemorrhagic) depending on the cause of the stroke. Ischemic strokes comprise the majority of strokes that occur as 85 percent of all strokes occurring because due to this condition. When an ischemic stroke occurs, the blood vessels are blocked by blood.

plaques, clusters, or greasy stores, dramatically diminuting the flow of oxygen and blood to the cerebrum or eliminating the mind's supply completely. A hemorrhagic brain stroke happens when a vein inside the cerebrum ruptures or explodes and causes a loss of blood flow to the brain. Both strokes, although distinct but are deadly in the same way and can be prevented by taking the same methods.

Factors Contributing to the Effect

The National Stroke Association has illustrated numerous factors that could easily and in a tangential manner contribute to the suffering of having a stroke. A poor eating pattern and latency, hypertension, elevated cholesterol, cardiovascular disease and diabetes all contribute to the prevalence of strokes. A better-planned diet with the best supplements, and a greater understanding with the health of one's body and the proven benefits of aloe Vera may increase the chances of avoiding the risk of having a stroke. An easy addition of 1-3 tablespoons of aloe vera in your daily schedule can positively impact the functioning of the mind and body, helping in limiting the chances of increasing the risk causes of strokes.

The most frequently described symptom of a stroke is the malfunctioning of the brain. the majority of patients who suffer from stroke say that their first sign something was not right was the inability to comprehend or communicate or experience a sudden sensation of paralysis or numbness the face or on the opposite part of their body.

Cancer

Cancer is defined as the sporadic growth of a variety of cells within the body. Sometimes referred to as threatening cells these dangerous changes on a phone level could occur in any tissue throughout the body. Invading every part of the body from the skin to bone, from the brain, the heart and every organ within your body. Cancerous cells may expand and grow quickly, and even metastasizing from one organ location to another in rapid in a series of. As a majority of malignant growths are not symptomatic (giving no evidence or signs that indicate the presence of disease) many patients do not realize they are suffering from malignant growths until the latest stage is reached. Early detection of the disease is the most effective aspect of treating malignant growth.

The reasons behind malignant growth could be different from the types of cancers. A staggering number of the factors to which people have been discovering for years are now considered to be risky diseases that don't only contribute to carcinogenic changes that occur at the level of cells, but also increase the rate of malignant growth and spreading. Exposure to sunlight as well as poisons like cigarette smoke and alcohol have been linked to the increase in cancer. Additionally, pre-existing ailments such as diabetes and obesity are also considered likely contributors to the development of this cancer.

Because each and every danger associated to the development of cancers (beside the genetic inclination) is dependent on a the right or wrong lifestyle choices, a growing number of physicians have turned their attention to developing their "counteraction is the most effective treatment" approach to reduce the incidence of cancer.

Many claim to have discovered an effective treatment for cancer. While research continues in the field, the September 2012 issue of BIOMEDICINE included a study by Shu-Chun Hsu , who described the efficacy of the emodin (an aloe

anthraquinone) in the deterrent of the growth of cancerous tumor cells. For more details about this research, please refer to the citation included in the appendix.

Debate Over Cancer Treatment Cancer Treatment Debate

When it comes to therapy is concerned, there is a vast range of assessments. Certain experts in clinical medicine suggest comprehensive strategies to kill malignant growth treatments, while others suggest the way of life and sustenance modifications. The most widely used treatments for diseases such as radiation and chemotherapy have long been seen as the best treatments to reestablish malignant growth. However, they have transformed into the source of heated discussions in recent months due to the fact that they are effective in identifying and killing malignant cells, yet they also kill solid cell. Solid cells' support is essential to the treatment, prevention and recovery processes that are associated as malignant growth. Without these cells the body is found to be more susceptible to disease, contamination and weird changes, resulting in a"powerful coincidence" circumstance that could result in the appearance of malignant growth or even worse.

People who promote nutrition-based treatment strategies can take an important place in the field of the medication referred to as elective medicine. There are a variety of studies that show specific medical benefits to the use of minerals and nutrients, similar to phytochemicals, people who advocate for elective medicine increase the use of nutrients to treat and prevent the onset of illness. Utilizing these common supplements for the body, many believe that the supplements and cell-building substances provided by aloe-vera could provide aids to malignant cells to shrink in size and quantity, and increasing the number of sound cells and aid in the overall functioning of the framework of safety (keeping up with solid susceptibility and overall health as well as receiving treatment). Experts in alternative medicine believe that due to the fact that carcinogenic cells are small and destroyed, while solid frameworks and cells benefit from improved well-being, the normal methods to monitor supplements as part of treatments for diseases should be looked at more closely.

How Aloe can help during treatment?

With its remarkable arrangement of normal Cell reinforcements the aloe-vera nutrients A C, A, and E and the naturally occurring sterols and other compounds, work to directly enhance cell health. this antioxidant support is the basis for the idea that is generating scientific research that investigate possibilities that aloe may be a beneficial treatment for cancer through reducing

detrimental changes and working to improve the amount of sound cells as well as the viability in the white blood platelets. The incredible sterile specialists of aloe help cells that are reinforced by limiting the health-destroying components in tissues and blood, working on general wellbeing and simultaneously limit the responsibility of the reparative cells needed to counteract harmful changes. The need to maintain a solid, immune-suppressed framework is crucial when the body's defenses are weak due to the effects of destructive changes. the ability of aloe vera to move through the motions of an antibacterial an antifungal, antiviral, and antimicrobial specialist could assist in defending against dangerous aggravations, delaying the burden of the resilient structure and allowing the safe framework to focus completely on carcinogenic areas and areas that aren't in good health. In the end the amino acids and other compounds that are found in aloe vera combine to aid those suffering from malignant tumors keep their energy levels up as well as a proper chemical equilibrium and efficient handling of supplements. will assist the entire body in functioning efficiently.

Aloe vera could also be a beneficial treatment for the secondary effects that can occur due to chemotherapy drugs and radiation therapy utilized to destroy harmful cells due to its proven ability to deal with radiation-related consumes. Additionally, aloe can be a powerful aid for treating stomach related issues and signs, and could help patients suffering from malignant growth by reducing some of the weakening secondary effects that result from cancer treatments.

Diabetes

Diabetes is a condition in which the body is unable to produce enough insulin, bringing the glucose level to an inexplicably high level in blood. Although this definition may seem a little naive, the affliction can be devastating and cost one American the life of a person on a regular basis. According to the World Health not really set as a fact that more than of 382 million people across the globe, suffer the negative effects of diabetes. Furthermore, the number of Americans who are battling the disease has risen by 40 percent to 29 million in only 10 years. In addition to killing more than AIDS and bosom malignant growth with the deaths attributed to diabetes account for a small part of the devastating consequences caused through the illness as the principal cause of eliminations (not due to injuries) and visual impairment kidney failure, cardiovascular breakdown and stroke, it is a major threat to daily life, but also causes a slow decline in the lives of diabetics. A typical double-up of patients with diabetes continuously until by 2030, the disease has evolved into a major concern, in the moment, but it will be the future of the population as well.

Diabetes is a condition that results from an incredibly impaired level of glucose or glucose, within the circulatory system, resulting due to the body's inability to effectively manage glucose. When you take a meal, your body transforms the food you eat into glucose which is a type of sugar utilized to create energy in cells. The glucose signals a response in the pancreas that triggers the release of insulin. The three different types of diabetes are type 1 type 1, type 2 and gestational.

Type 1 Diabetes

In addition, it is known as insulin-subordinate diabetes one diabetes can be described as an immune system issue that causes the body to perceive pancreatic cells as unwelcome intruders and attack them, in this way suppressing the body's production of insulin as well as the processing of glucose. Pancreatic cells that have been destroyed known as islets are accountable for detecting glucose and generating an important quantity of insulin. At the time that the insulin needs to be injected to the circulatory system the pancreatic cells that have been destroyed do not produce enough insulin or don't produce any insulin in any way. The faulty cycle prevents the cells of the body from accumulating the energy-producing glucose due to the fact that the insulin required to facilitate the process isn't available. The inability of cells to accept glucose results in an explosive domino effect that occurs when cells are unable to receive glucose, they become starving but they also leave naturally occurring glucose within the circulation system. This brings an increase in blood glucose levels or elevated glucose levels.

Type 2 Diabetes

It is a type of 2 diabetes is also referred to as being insulin-safe. This kind of diabetes usually occurs in people who are getting older and is the reason for the choice of adulthood and the beginning of diabetes. However, the number of adolescents and young people are developing this kind of diabetes. Type 2 diabetes means that it is evident that the amount of insulin released is insufficient for handling glucose. This is due to liver, muscle and fat cells that are perfectly, and not able to make use of insulin to transport glucose. The pancreas provides more insulin in order to pay back in the beginning, but fails to remain aware of requests for insulin or eventually requires help via medication as well as insulin injections.

Gestational Diabetes

Gestational diabetes is the type of diabetes that develops during pregnancy due to the explicit chemicals released during pregnancy, which cause insulin resistant. The condition typically disappears after the delivery of the baby gestational diabetes may trigger confusion during pregnancy and is often regarded as a precursor to the progression the condition of diabetes type 2 later on in the life.

How Aloe Can Help?

Due to the massive amount of minerals and nutrients within it, aloe vera helps in reducing the incidence of diabetes and its manifestations. The most beneficial aspect of aloe lies in its extraordinary phytochemicals. The two main issues that are associated by those suffering from diabetes are the components in the blood which are adversely affected by the excessive blood glucose, and also the inability to fully recover from an illness. The most widely accepted daily amount of consumption of aloe is about three tablespoons. Through the regular use of 1/3 of the daily day amount, several times every day, a person with diabetes could be able to bring back blood sugar levels to normal levels and have more consistent levels that are balanced for all day. In the form of a cream, aloe vera may be applied to diabetics' injuries as often as is necessary and in a quantity that will treat the injury in full. Because of its effectiveness in reducing glucose levels it is recommended that aloe vera not be eaten in conjunction with diabetic medications without first discussing the use of aloe vera in consultation with your doctor.

Aloe vera isn't just prepared to help in regaining time through ingested gel and application to the skin in the event of an issue with the body It can also help in the fight against the harmful levels of cholesterol, glucose, lipids, as well as fat oils that result from the ill-planned functioning of the pancreas and its related cells. By reducing, enhancing cell growth and glucose control properties Aloe vera can provide aloe-explicit catalysts that are accommodating and, in general, increases the amount of phytosterols, which help to reduce levels of bad cholesterol (LDL) and further increase the levels of cholesterol that is good (HDL) and manage blood pressure.

sugar levels and decrease the amount of lipids and other fatty substances in blood.

Obesity

In 2010 The Centers for Disease Control and Prevention released a report that contained shocking figures over 1/3 of American adult population was lean and 20 percent of children between the ages of between two and nineteen were obese. The report is described as an unfavorable aggregation of an exorbitant fat-to-muscle ratio, weight isn't just an aesthetic condition that creates restrictions, but a serious disease that could trigger more serious problems. With the number of obese people growing each year and that's only the beginning, and with more children getting fat, the need to be aware of the factors that contribute to it and the possibility of emerging conditions is evident in a way that has never been before. It's not a fact that the heftiness and related medical expenses have risen to $190.2 million, more than 21 percent of the total medical expenditures in America and the World Health Organization (WHO) as well as the Centers for Disease Control and Prevention (CDC) have recalled robustness in their plans of chronic diseases that plague America and the globe in general.

Obesity doesn't mean that it is an illness it is a condition that can be controlled and aggravated in the present. After some time of lifestyle decisions that contribute to the development of fat versus muscle and weight gain, obesity takes hold of the entire body. Through a lack of control over diet and a sedentary style of living, bizarre relaxation plans, the widespread use of drugs, alcohol and smoking contributing to the growth of the the ratio of fat to muscle and stoutness is a result of a deadly mix of lifestyle choices and inclinations. The most widely accepted measure of the heftiness of a person is the assessment from the data on weight (BMI) to determine if an individual is more than of 20% above what is considered"ordinary" for his height.

Body Mass Index (BMI)

The most commonly used calculation that is used to determine a person's weight is called the weight file (BMI) that is calculated by dividing the weight of a person in kilograms from the height in meters squared. By calculating the result the person will be able to identify the wording of

scheduled classes that span from being overweight to extremely obese.

For example, someone measuring 120 pounds and 5'6" tall will use the following calculation to calculate her BMI

1. Convert pounds into kilograms 120 times .453 = 54.43

2. Convert crawls into meters 5'6" (66") (66") x .0254 = 1.68

3. Square the change in metric that is subsequently made: $1.68^2 = 2.82$

4. Divide weight in kilograms by the height measured in meters 54.43/2.82 = 19.3

The subsequent estimate of 19.3 will then be used to decide the class of the weight territory which includes all BMI calculations starting at 18.5 to 40:

Weight is defined as less than 18.5

Normal: 18.5 -24.9

Overweight: 25 -29.9

Obese (class I) 30 -34.9

Obesity (class II) 35 -39.9

Very obese (class III) 40 or more

The Impacts of Obesity

Inflicting harm on the body's sequence of activities, events and structures, stoutness can unleash damage to the body through reducing the ability of the body's regular cycles and contributing to the development of real sicknesses and illnesses. Because of the size, many real-life conditions can develop that are aggravated by the hefty burden of the person.

The problems that are easily associated with excess weight have a clear correlation with the presence of bad cholesterol (LDL) as well as low levels of healthy cholesterol (HDL) hypertension, coronary illnesses metabolic disorder and malignant growth, stroke, joint pain, respiratory infections and aggravation. It can also lead to skin issues. As the onset of these conditions, obesity is not only a limitation of one's abilities and adversely affects one's satisfaction, but also creates a remarkable confluence of signs and symptoms which can lead to death.

How Aloe can help?

With the numerous benefits that aloe has on the cerebrum, blood organs, and the overall large-scale framework functioning within the organism, it's not surprising that aloe may assist in reducing the incidence of stoutness and its associated issues when used as a protective procedure, treatment or in the recovery interaction. Regarding fat and excessive weight gain is concerned, aloe may help by helping the body's digestion by limiting the development in fat cell, reducing the body's tendency for fat storage, as well as also enhancing the body's ability to build and maintain the muscle mass.

By arranging its essential amino acids and supplements it helps improve the body's ability to handle protein and fat, focusing on the body's ability to combine protein (working of muscles) while reducing the need for the elimination of fat. Aloe vera also plays an important role in cleansing organs and blood from fats and lipids that increase the quantity of fat within cells and in the courses. In addition to cleansing the blood of undesirable substances and toxins, the effects of aloe vera on the cardiovascular system can also help in regulating sugar levels and reducing the risk of developing diabetes, which is a condition that usually is caused by overweight.

Aloe vera is able to fight weight by providing essential phytochemicals and supplements that can influence diet, exercise rest, and chemical production. With an abundance of nutrients, minerals along with amino acids aloe is able to help in the area of diet, improving the functioning of the body's systems and reducing insufficiencies that contribute to an increase in weight and fatigue. The phytochemicals and protein that aloe has also aid in stopping rest patterns and chemical production, delivering some sort of calming effect which can help you avoid falling asleep and staying awake. The components of aloe can lessen the adverse consequences on weight that outcome from absence of rest and sporadic rest designs, in particular the over the top creation of cortisol (a weight-gaincontributing chemical) and an expanded needing for sugars. In addition, with the advantages of aloe's cell bolsters that protect the fragile framework from threats that can affect health and worsen existing health issues Aloe vera is proven to be among the most effective options to an exercise routine that is expected to reduce the amount of weight you gain. By adding the typical daily dose of three tablespoons of aloe to your daily diet will help you work on the various capacities that are associated with weight loss as well as executive maintenance.

Recipes

Blueberry-Banana Breakfast Smoothie

This smoothie is a fantastic choice for any heart-healthy eating regimen. It's packed with cell support and protein and amino acids, potassium as well as nutrient C to rid the blood of toxins, reduce circulation, and keep

keep your glucose levels in check up, and protect yourself from illness and diseases.

Ingredients Serves 2

1/4 CUP ALOE VERA JUICE

1/4 CUP CRUDE OATS ROLLED

2 cups almond milk unsweetened

1/2 CUP FROZEN BLUEBRIES

One medium-sized banana sliced and frozen

1. Mix oats and aloe vera in a blender and blend until the oats have mixed.

2. Mix in the remaining fixings until the fixatives are mixed.

Almond-Blueberry Freeze

This sugar-balancing smoothie prevents diabetic issues, and improves general wellbeing as well.

INGREDIENTS

SERVES 2

1/4 cup aloe vera juice

1/2 cup of normal, crude almonds, unsalted 11/2 cups

unsweetened almond milk 1 Cup plain Greek yogurt

1/2 cup frozen blueberries

1. Mix almonds and aloe vera in a blender, then mix until the almonds have blended.

2. Mix the remaining fixings in until the fixatives are mixed.

Sweet Green Smoothie

It is a good idea to supplement your diet with thick vegetables. organic food products, which are combined with cancer prevention agents green tea, rich in antioxidants to help to achieve and maintain the best health for any stage of life.

Ingredients

Serves 2

1/4 CUP ALOE VERA JUICE

2 cups green tea that has been fermented and chilled

1/2 cup slashed spinach

3/4 medium pear sliced and cored

1 medium banana de-stemmed and frozen

1/2 cup frozen blueberries

Mix all ingredients in blender. Mix until smooth.

Pumpkin Pie Smoothie

Smoothies that are rich with nutrient A may help in further improving eye health. Nutrient A is especially important to prevent Glaucoma as you get older.

Ingredients

Serves 2

1/4 cup aloe vera juice

Half cup of pure pumpkin

1/2 medium yam, cooked and stripped 2 cups of unsweetened vanilla almond milk one teaspoon crushed cinnamon

Ground cloves, 1/2 teaspoon

Combine all the fixings in the blender. Mix until smooth.

Berry-Banana Shake

The vibrant color of berries comes from the anthocyanins' high concentrations which provide incredible protection against infection and sickness. Due to the growth of aloe, and the addition of the supplement of food that is thick this drink takes the health benefits of berries to an unprecedented of height, alleviating breathing problems and other conditions.

Ingredients

Serves 2

1/4 CUP ALOE VERA JUICE

2 cups almond milk that is unsweetened, vanilla and unsweetened

1/2 CUP BLACKBERRIES

1/2 CUP RASPBERRIES

1 large banana de-stemmed and frozen

Mix all ingredients in the blender. Mix until smooth.

Chapter 10: Inflammation

Many people are aware of the possibility of aggravation, they are prone to think about joint discomfort. Although it is true that joint discomfort can become a normal problem that is caused by constant aggravation, it's certainly not the only (or often the only) situation that's associated by irritation. The process of irritation is used by the invulnerable frame to heal the body properly but when the normal cycle is disrupted, the consequences are aplenty across the body, and medical issues can cause. Aloe vera is a natural remedy that can be a significant factor in reducing your frequency as well as its impact.

How does inflammation manifest?

It is not an entirely understood component of infection, since specialists are still unsure of the exact causes of irritation. The idea of irritation is that it is an appropriate reaction, but it remains in "on" phase. For a normal, sound person it is the body's reaction to the opposite side of the frame; in a patient who suffers from chronic aggravation the body's response to the injury continues to be initiated, leading to irritation, sickness and even disease.

blood tests that serve as indicators to determine whether a person is who are suffering from chronic or acute inflammation or predisposed to develop inflammation. There are a few tests available the majority of people suffering from inflammation depend on self-observations and diagnosis from doctors familiar with inflammatory disorders.

If you are suffering from the negative effects of an infection or injury, your body's response is to start the healing process as fast as is reasonable and then support the recuperating cycle until the body is back to its normal state. In the event of an injury or disease the body sends a positive signal to the fiery specialists, which signal the white plates to initiate the healing process. This part of the process is often referred by some as an aggravation process can be seen in real-time by the redness, pain expanding, heat, and redness. The white platelets then work to eliminate the contaminant and damaged tissues, while the mitigating process intensifies to complete the healing process.

In the case of a fiery illness or condition in which the explosive mixtures that support it does not stop which results in constant aggravation to the space or framework affected. The constant agitation causes an unintended domino result of malfunctioning cells and organ systems that may eventually develop into severe inflammatory disorders that do not just affect the quality of life, but also can result in more serious illnesses.

Different types of inflammation

Inflammation can trigger intense discomfort within a specific area, or it can develop into an all-encompassing issue that afflicts at the very least an individual of our structures. Since it's hard to determine, the issue could progress in the long run and eventually become the primary cause for a more serious problem. It is able to affect every cell or tissue in the body, inflammation has been identified as the primary reason behind many common illnesses. Although the article isn't long it does not cover the unavoidable effects that stress creates throughout the body, with no focus on the specific area.

Rheumatoid arthritis is inflammation of the joints as well as the tissues that surround joints

Ankylosing spondylitisis an inflammation of the vertebrae ligaments, muscles and the sacroiliac joints

Celiac disease is an swelling of the small intestinal tract

Crohn's disease is an inflammation of the digestive tract

Fibromyalgia is an irritation of the nerves as well as various body parts

Graves" disease is an inflammation of the thyroid gland

Idiopathic Pulmonary Fibrosis: inflammation in the alveoli inside the lung.

Lupus Inflammation of joints the lungs, joints kidney, skin, and joints.

Psoriasis is inflammation of the skin

Sinusitis is sinus inflammation

Allergies: inflammation of different areas of the body

When irritation begins in a single point and affecting just one area in the body. spreading of the problem can lead to different areas being affected by the ongoing issue that quickly transforms into a illness. The nerves, joints muscles, tendons digestive tract and bones, the aggravation could create severe limitations on the body's normal working and processes.

Inducing stiff joints, weak energies, inadequate absorption skin issues, and continuous discomfort throughout the body, irritation could adversely affect your personal satisfaction. What's more painful than feeling a little irritation in extreme instances is the possibility of the irritation becoming unending. If the irritation in one area is spread to anotherarea, the intense gets worse and persistent an illness. The development of coronary disease, tumors, and other dangerous illnesses can arise from irritation. The medications available for clinical use rarely offer relief or reverse the symptoms. This is reason why prevention could be the best option to carry on living your life without suffering, and this is that aloe can help.

Aloe's protein 14kDa in size, was thoroughly studied in an

Recent study in 2010 conducted by Swagata Das from India following lengthy isolating and presenting the protein to certain illnesses the researchers concluded that the aloespecific protein as effective against inflammation and fungi in the body. For more information, click here.

Information, please refer to the study's information in Appendix B.

Common Treatments

Inflammation can affect every part of the body and may spread quickly to various structures and parts. Since irritation is the root of all these ailments and diseases It's not a surprise that billions of dollars are used each year to treat. As everyone is susceptible to the possibility of suffering from a physical problem or some sort of contamination at some point in their life, the risk of causing irritation is real. The ailment of aggravation is a common response in everyone, therefore, the most dreadful outcome that could be conceivable of experiencing an irritation path that does not "turn off" is one that can affect anyone at any time. That's why there is a recommendation from the World Health Organization recommends that combating the symptoms could be the best method of treatment.

The majority of anti-microbials and medications offer the same risks and benefits. Nonsteroidal mitigating medications (NSAIDs) can be described as the most frequently employed calming medicine of decision. Although these medications are available in the form of a prescription but they also have a wide range of potentially harmful incidental consequences. Acetaminophen is additionally used to treat pain and fever, but could also contribute to many difficult problems resulting from abuse. The meds prescribed by a physician that stop the cyclooxygenase protein that causes irritation as well as fever and pain may be beneficial and feasible at the moment however, they have been linked with a higher risk of heart disease and stroke.

There is an increasing number of doctors who are vocal in their efforts to educate consumers about the risks of repeated or overuse of antibiotics. The immune system is weakening which can cause adverse reactions in the body and in its systems and causing

an environment where new and more severe illnesses could cause havoc, doctors are urging the public to use antibiotics only as an option last resort.

Being aware that the need for aggravation is vital to a typical recuperation process, it is reasonable to believe that the root of the problem is in the normal functioning in the body. As we have seen the adverse effects of the commonly approved drug drugs, many experts in the health and wellness field are now examining the drugs and recommending a more effective way of preventing and treating this common occurrence may lie in the routine procedures.

Aloe vera is now in focus as a remedy for inflammation due to its ability to naturally reduce inflammation, while improving the health of your body's cells and systems as well as improving the function of the immune system (the cause in inflammation). With no adverse side negative effects, like the effects of laxatives that many people who use aloe are familiar, aloe offers proved benefits that are greater than risk. With a growing amount of research revealing the results of drugs treatment, the aloe-vera method is gaining popularity.

How Aloe can help?

Natural wellness professionals have started applying a regular treatment method that focuses on the root of irritation, which is usually. After observing the negative effects of a lack of exercise and stress, rest and other lifestyle causes that lead to things and the persistence of the aggravation growing, more medical professionals and doctors have switched towards more standard mending methods that take the entire body and its structures into account.

In the January 2014 edition of CARBOHYDRATE POLYMERS, Dr. Min-Cheol Kang effectively proved the aloe vera polysaccharides' (APS) free-radical-scavenging capabilities and their ability to fight off oxidative stress caused by free radicals and inflammation. For more details on the research, and ways to learn more, look up Appendix B.

Due to the frustration of "not having a clear understanding of" the causes, effects and necessity of treatment for irritation, the medical local region has joined the regular experts in identifying the conditions of being commonly encountered in patients suffering from aggravation. This increased attention to aspects that cause or cause inflammation, like factors in the diet and lifestyle factors, has resulted in an enormous amount of research which has revealed certain ailments that are typically associated with the diagnosis of inflammatory disorders. It is a good thing that this focus on the seemingly random ailments associated to irritation, along with a better understanding of the interaction within the body's structures could provide answers to the problem. As we shift our focus on the normal aspects of the process and final results happening in the body that experience irritation, the possibility that "normal ailments react to standard treatments" is now becoming more widely recognized for prevention and treatment of irritation.

in the INTERNATIONAL JOURNAL of PHARMACEUTICS Issue 333, March 2007, there was research paper, "Skin permeation enhancement potential of Aloe Vera" and a proposal for

mechanism of action that is based on the pull and size effect" It was discovered that aloe vera , not only penetrates skin more effectively than comparable products however it also enhances the capability of the products getting into the skin, when used together.

When aloe was initially controlled to treat skin disorders and the gastrointestinal system and gastrointestinal framework, the results were successful. The result was subsequently accompanied by the use of aloe that prompted studies of the use of aloe across various health areas. As time progressed and treatment methods developed, it wasn't really established in stone that the usual phytochemicals present in aloe offer cancer-prevention agent as well as antimicrobial, sterile and some mitigating effects. These phytochemicals, made up of several nutrients, enzymes, as well as specific phytochemicals that are aloe-specific, proved to be beneficial in treating at the time, and continue be beneficial today. The body is hydrated and sustenance, as well as providing support and protection, aloe vera is proven to be effective in a variety of areas of health especially when it comes to irritation. Through limiting the effects of aloe on an aggressor and the benefits it offers, aloe's naturally occurring soothing phytochemicals can aid in the healing process and can work on different mechanisms and capacities that contribute to the escalating events and the persistence of aggravation. Research has been conducted to determine the efficacy of the anti-inflammatory properties of aloe vera across every part of the body, ranging from the digestive system to the skin, to hemorrhoids and specific organs. The results from these studies have revealed that aloe vera is a great way to aid in the healing process of inflammation and decrease the risk of inflammation in all parts of the body. For specific information about studies regarding aloe and its impact on inflammation, refer to the appendices.

Amino Acids

It provides an astonishing Twenty of the amino acids necessary to function properly in the framework of the entire body, aloe vera is able to minimize the risks and events of aggravation.

With adequate amounts of amino acids our body's structures are supported however, the function improves as does the susceptibility to infection and the two main elements of aggravation are largely eliminated. With arginineand isoleucine as well as leucine and phenylalanine circulating around as remarkable mitigating specialists Aloe vera provides massive amounts of potent supplements which reduce the severity of existing discomfort, but also help to prevent irritation from causing. By taking a daily portion of the recommended 3-4 tablespoons of aloe you can dramatically improve their intake of amino acids and reap the benefits associated with their entry and absorption.

To make the experience even more, the pain that is the reason that a lot of people resort to remedies and over-the-counter medications to control is addressed effectively and usually through these amino acids, with a few often becoming more effective in relieving discomfort than the usual medications used. In addition to ensuring a safe and secure environment the twenty amino acids do not only assist in improving circulation of blood through cardiovascular aid however, they also work to rid the blood of toxins and protect the body from illnesses caused by microorganisms infections and growths as well as microorganisms. These might be hesitant about a resistance to the framework and could result in a long-lasting cycle of inflammation.

Vitamins

An array of nutrients can be found in aloe vera. The nutrients A, C, E K, as well as all the essential Bs work within the body to aid the frameworks and organs by making sure that they function properly. As you are likely to be aware, a nutrient deficiency could cause a decline in the performance of a framework, resulting in an impact that cascades on the frameworks that depend on the negatively impacted one. Vitamins A, C as well as E, have been proven to enhance the framework's well-being by virtue of their cells' reinforcement properties that help strengthen the body's resistive structure while sustaining the normal functioning of the body's system.

Vitamin An insufficiency is a common condition among aggravation victims, regardless of an impact or cause in addressing the nutritional An insufficiency has been proven to alleviate the symptoms of irritation and reduce the discomfort and adverse negative effects that can result. Aloe vera is a source of the nutrient A, but also helps to ensure the body's intake of nutrient A. It does this by providing different minerals that assist in the process of handling and utilizing the nutrients A, C and E.

Minerals

As a powerful supporting components that perform multiple functions minerals fulfill twofold duty by assisting the body's normal functioning as well as incredible electrolytes that boost the health of stomach, blood, chemicals and levels of liquids throughout the body. With an array of vital minerals such as magnesium, iron as well as zinc, copper, and iron that are able to influence the balance of chemicals and blood's health as well as the functioning of the cardiovascular system It's no surprise that the aloe's minerals help in the reduction of inflammation.

In charge of delivering the most essential nutrients to the body's organs and structures, the blood's main components, white platelets, red plateslets and plasma, can also easily trigger aggravation. The subsequent the initiation of, also known as "bringing the inflow" from white plates towards the location of a physical problem or contamination is among the most beneficial factors of aggravation. This is enhanced when the necessary minerals help to keep up with the proper functioning and guidelines of white platelets. The next stage of the incendiary cycle is chemicals that are beneficial to provocative specialists that are then interacting and causing constant irritation. The copper and zinc that aid in managing these chemicals are abundant in aloe. They work on the development and use of stimulating and reducing chemicals. Aloe vera reduces the risky work that results in the"aggravation course" of these hormones.

Particular phytochemicals

Aloe is unique because it contains potent phytochemicals that function synergistically to enhance wellbeing and maintain the normal functions of the body as well as its structure. The phytochemicals aid in the treatment of provocative conditions by reducing irritation, minimizing the discomfort associated with flaming symptoms and helping to recover tissue that is lost due to delayed continuous inflammation.

One of these naturally occurring substances, lipase is a substance that aids aloe to penetrate the skin's various layers, when applied topically enhancing the antioxidant and calming effects on the rest of the body, allowing these effects to enter the blood supply, and consequently, all the organs which are supplied by blood.

In reducing the discomfort of all regions affected by inflammation, the sterols in plants, such as beta-sitosterol, lupeol, and campesterol work directly at the point of inflammation, with powerful anti-inflammatory properties. These effects do not just apply to the region of discomfort however they are distributed across the body to find and eliminate the agents that cause inflammation in the bloodstream. Reducing the discomfort that occurs due to aroused areas of the body, aloe's salicylic acid offers a headache medication-like benefit that eases symptoms of pain through suppressing the release of prostaglandin chemical compounds that cause discomfort and an agony reaction within nerves. The aggravation-freeing perspective of aloe is evident due to the fact that it contains a commonly present catalyst, bradykinin which aids in breaking the amazing agony messengers that transmit to the body and brain.

The most intriguing phytochemicals provided by aloe vera as treatment and anticipation of irritation are the polysaccharides that assist the tissues that have been damaged or destroyed in the time of continual irritation, rebuild and recover, bringing relief from irritation by creating new tissues and cells. The generally recommended daily dose of 1-3 tablespoons aloe vera has been proven beneficial effects in the reduction of irritation and it is possible to improve the results with efficient applications too. Applying a generous amount of aloe vera on the areas that are irritated on the body, you will be able to reduce irritation and discomfort topically whenever it is necessary.

Recipes

Amazing Applesauce

The simple and quick fruit puree is clearly superior to the local variety. All-natural fixings reduce irritation within the body.

Ingredients

Serves 6

4 cups of water

Four medium-sized apples cut from their cores, chopped and cored

1 CUP ALOE VERA JUICE

1 tablespoon ground cinnamon

1. In a large stockpot, mix apples and water.

2. Make a bubbly over high heat. Reduce heat to low and cook for 30 to 45 minutes or until the apples are tender to the touch.

3. Blend the apples in blender and mix in cinnamon and aloe vera.

4. Blend on high until desired consistency is reached.

Apple-Berry Smoothie

You can satisfy your sweet tooth by drinking this delicious and relaxing drink which contains cancer prevention drugs to help reduce cell damage and the risk of developing. Ingredients

SERVES 2

1/4 cup aloe vera juice

2 cups almond milk unsweetened and unsweetened

1 medium-sized apple, cut, cored and

1. Cleaved 1 Cup frozen strawberries

1/8 CUP SWEET FLAXSEED GROUND

Combine all the fixings in the blender. Mix until smooth.

Tropical Refresher

This amazing combination of tropical flavors provides astonishing health benefits to every area of the body, reducing inflammation.

Ingredients Serves 2

1/4 CUP ALOE VERA JUICE 1/2 CUP

COCONUT OIL 11/2 CUPS WATER

2 cups cleaved , cleaved and cored pineapple removed and cored. Combine all ingredients in blender. Mix until smooth.

Simple Salsa

When food that is delicious is able to make positive changes in the body and body, it can make "eating to be healthy" easier! This incredible, mildly hot salsa is tasty and provides all the body with vitamins, minerals as well as amazing phytochemicals!

Ingredients

Serves 10

5 tiny Roma tomatoes Cored, slashed and slashed 2

cloves garlic, minced

1/4 cup cleaved cilantro 1/4 cup aloe

Vera juice 1/4 cup red onion diced 1/3 cup

Cup of diced celery

2 tablespoons lime juice

1. A medium-sized bowl is used to mix garlic, tomatoes and cilantro. mix to coat.

2. Make sure to join the rest of the fixings using an fork till all the fixings have been connected.

3. Keep it in the refrigerator for up to two days.

Roasted Turmeric Potatoes

Potatoes that are dense, anti-cancer agent turmeric and solid fats extracted from olive oil help to adjust glucose and a solid blood fat guidelines. This tasty side dish does more than provide relief for those who are prone to crashes and sugar surges however it also helps reduce chronic inflammation.

Ingredients serve 2

1/8 cup is added two tablespoons of olive oil

2 massive Idaho Baking potatoes sliced and cut into cubes 1 clove of garlic, chopped

1 teaspoon turmeric powder

Salt , pepper and as desired

1/4 cup aloe vera juice

1. Preheat the broiler to 400°F. Spread a large baking pan with two tablespoons of olive oil.

2. In a huge bowl, combine potatoes, remaining garlic, olive oil and turmeric. Spread potatoes on baking sheets and spread equally.

3. For 20 minutes, bake or until you can feel the delicate fork. Turn and continue baking for about 15 minutes or until all the potatoes are nicely cooked.

4. Remove broiler from oven then sprinkle on salt and black pepper. Let cool for five minutes before throwing aloe vera over the broiler to cover.

Chapter 11: Brain Health

The cerebrum is the largest and most complex organ in the entire body, responsible to the actions, messages and the functioning of every organ within the human body. It is supported by the various elements that affect the frameworks as well as the components which demonstrate to easily provide support for these frameworks, the brain is the main control system that all the aspects of the body are influenced. From the actions and responses to imagination and thought, it is the primary force to be reckoned with by the body and from where all commands are issued. For all the power it has but a brain's weakness can cause serious problems for the actual and psychological cycles we consider to be normal "everyday" capabilities. With the most current knowledge about the requirements and obligations that the brain has, we are able to find essential ways to enhance and sustain brain health and proper functioning of the mind. Aloe Vera is one of the benefits of a regular living that can provide substantial benefits in the direction of the mind, helping to reverse the damage and enhancing it over a long period of time to be.

The Introduction To Your Brain

The cerebrum is the most complex and amazing organ of the human body. The three-pound organ is divided in two parts of the world and comprises three main working areas as well as three flaps. There are numerous supporting structures that run around as correspondence conveyance frameworks between the cerebrum and the body (as as well as the other direction). Through a simple outline of the components of the brain and an in-depth description of each function, you'll better understand the synergy this organ has and the significance of keeping up with the health of the body's supporting structures to ensure proper functioning of the cerebrum.

entirety. With the plethora of brain-related responses happening throughout the cerebrum and in a logical way, an insignificant breakdown could cause major complications. Aversion to a particular course or the cascading effect observed in various parts of the body's health An issue with the cerebrum triggers an immediate concern of comparing parts of the body. This can result in the disintegration of actions or the absence of any correspondence.

Ability to control, manage and coordinate an astonishing amount of reactions, actions functions, processes and synergies within the system, the brain is comprised of interconnected components, supporting sub-sections, and vital components that work together to enable breathing, respiration digestion, movement and emotions feasible. If one part of the brain is affected, the rest of the brain will suffer, causing disturbances in memory, thought speech, behavior and learning, among others. Through being aware of the different brain regions and how each one plays a role in our everyday lives and functioning, you will better appreciate the importance of maintaining a healthy brain and the best ways to assist those areas in order to ensure and improve the functioning of your brain.

Two Hemispheres

The cerebrum can be divided by two sides of the equator: both sides. Each underlying component there's two sides, a left and right, which reflect each other and facilitating the functions of various organs within the human body. A surprising fact is that when the signals coming from cerebrums to bodies (as as well as the reverse ways around) transmit the body's messages, they confuse. In the final moment, left cerebrum and right body transmit, in the same way that the right cerebrum as well as the left body transmit as shown by a stroke patient who's suffered strokes on the left side of the brain and is unable to deal with the right half of their body and the reverse. The two halves of the planet are divided into three regions.

Three regions of the brain is located in various locations of the cerebrum. They control various aspects of normal capabilities, and interacts to different frameworks. The three regions of the brain are hindbrains, midbrains, and forebrain. They are responsible to the body's functioning through a variety of methods:

The hindbrain is situated behind the brain, and is comprised of the spinal cord's upper part as well as the brain stem and cerebellum. The hindbrain controls the body's functions, including breathing, pulse and processing, the essential parts of the body that do not require cognizant control.

The midbrain is located in the uppermost part of the brainstem this part regulates reflex actions and plays a role in voluntary actions such as eye movements.

The forebrain is the biggest and most developed part of the brain. It consists of the cerebrum, the thalamus and the hypothalamus. Also known as an "inner brain" the brain's forebrain process and uses information, and then relays this information back to brain as well as the body. The cerebral cortex comprises the area of the brain that is responsible for thinking, behavior, and actions. This is known as the cerebral cortex which is broken down into four distinct sections, referred to as lobes.

FOUR LOBES

The four lobes in the cerebral cortex are each responsible for distinct functions throughout the body. Processing information related to scents and sights as well as information and education memory formation, recognition of visuals and memory formation. These areas are the miniature control areas of the brain which are responsible for various aspects of our self. A single lobe's impact could completely alter a person's character, personality, abilities to talk, thinking processing and the ability to regulate physical functions. Because of their importance each of these lobes is extensively discussed as the functions of the brain are explained:

Frontal lobe is responsible for thinking, planning, imagination emotion, speech and problem-solving The frontal lobe is crucial to the creation of innovative ideas as well as heated debates.

Parietal lobe: located in front of the frontal lobe this area is responsible for recognizing of movement direction and processing information from the senses. The texture, taste and scents of an incredible food item are all produced there, as is the physical control that lets you cut food and then move it to your mouth by making complex movements of your fork, knife or spoon.

Occipital lobe: located between the eyes. The occipital region can be responsible for the processing of information from the visual. The splendor of autumn leaves the sunset, as well as rainbows are completely captured and interpreted by this lobe.

Temporal lobe: This lobe is responsible for emotion, perception and recognition, as well as auditory information processing, memory and speech. The song you heard at the age of eighteen and made you cry is preserved as a memory in this lobe.

Supporting Components

With all the activity in the brain that guides and sustaining every aspect of the human body, the parts that support the functioning of the cerebrum are essential. The neurons, cells, and neurotransmitters that comprise the core of the brain also serve as lines of communication between different cerebrum's cells and between the cerebrum as well as the body's structures.

When a malfunction occurs in only one of these support patterns, the entire body can be affected.

Neurons are tiny powerhouses that produce messages that are transmitted through neurotransmitters at speeds that are 400 miles an hour as well as from the other neuron "speaking" directly to body and brain about movement thoughts, feelings and memories. In and around the neuron are specific structures that do not only serve as a function for the neurons and its functions, but also aid in the communications between neurons as well as connections between the body and brain.

Cell body: including the nucleus The cell body produces energy molecules that support the neuron's functions.

Dendrites: growing like branches that extend from the body of the cell, the dendrites carry messages to cells.

Axons: extending beyond the cell just like dendrites do, Axons are accountable for transporting messages out of the body of cells. Axons are responsible for releases of neurotransmitters in the synapses, transferring messages to the receptors in the organs, cells, as well as systems.

Sheath: more than an outer layer of protection for neurons, the myelin sheath helps to improve the speed in message transmitting and reception. The promotion of health and well-being of the myelin sheath of the neuron makes sure that the maximum speed, which is believed to be around 400 miles/hour is achievable.

With all the components of each component being totally

dependent on each other being inextricably linked to see how simple weaknesses or breakdowns within the power of one part can cause devastating impact on the functioning of the entire body. The health of these supporting structures of the mind is vital to maintaining the well-being of the cerebrum and the health of the body that it gives. Research has shown that these regions of the mind thrive when they have sufficient oxygen and macronutrients, micronutrients as well as a steady amount of glucose.

Aloe's capacity to aid in maintaining and controlling the levels of glucose, and supply different minerals and nutrients needed for proper functioning and handling within cells, and improve the body's handling of cerebral oxygen flow, it's difficult to comprehend how the regular use of aloe could assist in maintaining the health of the brain's elements that directly affect the health that the brain is in.

Dysfunctions in the Brain

The National Institute of Neurological Disorders and Stroke has been the leader and supporter of many studies of the brain and how it functions every year. Since the 1990s , the amount of information about the cerebrum and its structure, as well as its capacities have become evident due to the endless analysis and studies across the globe. A large number of these studies have focused on the functioning of the cerebrum in general providing us with insights about the processes, demands, and co-operative relationships that the brain relies on to function at its peak. In contrast, a significant portion of these studies have focused focussed on the minds suffering from injuries, degeneration or illness, which bring problems in the brain's cycle. These breakdowns have been organized into categories that classify dysfunctions based on their purpose area of impact, their goal or the adverse effects that occur by the dysfunction

Neurogenetic: defective genes can be responsible for the creation of neurological diseases like

Huntington's disease as well as muscular dystrophy.

Developmental: during the process of developing the body can suffer from dysfunctions that can affect any part of the brain and spinal cord, resulting in disorders like spinal bifida.

As one gets older and deteriorates the brain's parts causes damage or death of nerve cells, which can lead to degenerative diseases such as Alzheimer's disease and Parkinson's disease.

Metabolic: because of a dysfunctional metabolic process the brain's functioning gets affected , resulting in diseases like Gaucher's Disease.

Cerebrovascular diseases that impact the blood vessels that supply the brain with the oxygen and blood cause problems with brain functioning and lead to diseases such as strokes , vascular dementia.

Trauma: a trauma to the spinal cord or brain can have a significant impact on the brain's function and nerves that aid in the connection between the body and brain. The paralysis example is only one instance of how injury to the spinal cord or the brain can result in total "disconnection" with the body and brain.

Epileptic and convulsive experiences cause seizures. the physical manifestations of the body and brain malfunctioning.

Infectious: viruses, bacteria and inflammation may severely affect the overall health and wellbeing of spinal cord and the brain leading to the development of infections and severe destruction to tissues and cells of nerves. AIDS and meningitis, dementia, and Encephalitis are just some of the conditions that arise from inflammation and infection within our nervous system.

The development of abnormal cells in the brain may hinder overall brain functioning , or are confined to a specific part within the brain. Due to the growth of cancerous cells cancer and tumors can destroy the brain's cells, causing the brain's dysfunction or even death.

Maintaining the health of your brain

Modern technology has enabled researchers to learn more about the cerebrum over the past twenty years, which is not the case at any other time. Through the use of symbols and perceptions the clinical locale is able to gain a better understanding of the brain's spaces and their capacities as well as dysfunctions as well as their needs. the

result of poor judgment. To maintain cerebrum health, a variety of life choices and exercises are a crucial aspect to cooperate simple ways to improve the strength of the mind, while also developing the strength of the frameworks that aid the brain to function properly. With diets, psychological exercise active work, diet and lifestyle choices that reduce the effects of stress, illness and aversion to harmful parts, the cerebrum will not only be able to function properly but it will grow!

Diet

With the countless areas and mental cycles that require various essential supplements in order to function properly It is essential to have a regular diet that provides the necessary nutrients in adequate amounts. The body requires amino acids and glucose, as well as minerals, nutrients, as well as cell-building substances from diet, every aspect and capability of the mind relies on the nutrition that is provided by diet. In the event of dietary deficiencies directly affecting mental health and the functioning of each part of the body, placing a greater emphasis on healthy food choices not only increases and sustains the vibrancy of the cerebrum but also the body as a whole.

Physical Exercise

" Moving bodies stay moving" is not just a reference to joints and muscles. When you are constantly captivated in physical activity the cerebrum body connection remains locked within. As you use it smartphones and frameworks which work in synergy to provide the development and transmit to and away, animate the synapses' firing and the more stimulants are added to the brain, the more it remains conditioned for responding and responding. When you working, the cerebrum releases endorphins which produce sensations of energy and improve generally positive disposition. These feelings lead to a more evident desire for well-being, enhancing the possibility of engaging in the actual workplace and maintaining the pattern of progressed with good habits that contribute to the power of the mind as well as the body.

Lifestyle Choices

The reason could be tension or an openness to risky environmental elements the cerebrum makes certain ways of making life decisions. Being open to components that are antagonistic to it like mercury and aluminum (just to mention a few of harmful components that are incalculably harmful) can influence the brain's components and cycles, which can impede the natural cycles that occur in the cerebrum as well as the body. With the growing amount of evidence on the impact that weight has on our minds, it's widely accepted that injuries and other circumstances that create stress on the mind can affect how it thinks but they also have the capability to harm brain's underlying structures. Possible outcomes include an increase in the hormone production, weakened processes involved in communication, as well as the growth of serious illness and illnesses, life-style factors which expose the brain and body to negative elements (both psychological and physical) must be eliminated to ensure the health of the brain.

How Aloe can help?

Since the beginning of time aloe has been used for treating ailments, but at no point were there any data available with the ways that aloe could help with working process and maintain the mental strength. Through innumerable studies and exploration aloe has been proven to provide significant enhancements across the body, and in particular the mind. Through its arrangement of vital nutrients needed in the cerebrum aloe is able to protect the various parts of our mind's cycles and the connection to every cell and structure in the human body. With specific phytochemicals to assist with fighting sickness, fight irritation, and cleanse your bloodstream, it safeguards the health of the cerebrum but is also able to safeguard the foundations upon the foundations on which it is based.

Glucose

Dependent on a constant amount of glucose that is readily available and the mind's incredibly metabolic capabilities and cycles are dependent on the body's capability to provide and control the amount of glucose that is in blood. The cells are supplied with fuel they need to produce energy and energy, glucose directly affects the functioning of the brain.

of synapses' when cells are functioning properly of the synapses, the brain can produce numerous responses that occur every second, making the actual development thoughts, musings and emotions possible. When glucose is not readily available or hypoglycemia, the cerebrum experience changes at a cell level which can cause a lack of concentration, a decrease in responses and fatigue.

Aloe assists in the handling and guiding of glucose, not only through its ability to regulate blood sugar levels but also by providing the different supplements required to make use of glucose, and making it available to phone for use. With B-nutrients amino acids, B vitamins, and all the minerals necessary to handle glucose, aloe is a simple way to improve the functioning of the synapses' as well as the cycle in which they are involved.

Amino Acids

The amino acids that are activated every time a response is made in the body are most needed within the brain. To create and strengthen the synapses, which are responsible to transmit the huge amount of messages that are sent to and from those synapses, the brain requires plenty of amino acids.

With 20 amino acids out of 22, the aloe plant can assure that the cerebrum has the amino acids that are essential to create new synapses and to keep pace with the strength of the existing ones. Additionally, in support of the use of amino acids in the development of synapses. Aloe's steady zinc supplements ensure that the handling of amino acids is accurate and improves the functioning of synapses that have been recently integrated that result out of this process.

Vitamins

Aloe provides the body with all the essential B nutrients that aid the brain develop of myelin, the sheath which is the brain's protective cover. This protective covering assists in ensuring the rapid occurrence of compound responses as well as the speedy transmission of electrical impulses both the mind and body are dependent on the structure of this vital cover. Aloe vera's extraordinary combination of the minerals (it is the primary plant that has B12) assures the character that the sheath of myelin is responsible for its development and growth.

A further B nutrient essential to be found by aloe is the thiamin that is utilized by the cerebrum in order to keep up with the synapses' layers and to improve the nerves' conductivity. A further benefit of aloe's B-nutrients are the guideline resulting from a process of amino corrosive digestion , also known as homocysteine. By providing B6, B12 as well as folate, which are essential to regulate homocysteine levels, it helps prevent cerebrum degeneration , which causes issues such as Alzheimer's and intellectual break-down caused by high levels of homocysteine.

Similar to the B nutrients are essential to the brain, which requires large quantities of nutrientC to create the norepinephrine which is an synapse. This nutrient isn't just that is found in aloe, but the many minerals present in aloe also assist in increasing the intake of nutrient C. This makes it more quickly available to the brain.

Minerals

Minerals are used by the cerebrum, but not only to assist in the formation and development of its components but also as powerful supplements that aid in supporting. Enhancing the functioning of synapses' as well as those synapses which transmit messages between them, the minerals are essential in keeping pace with the power of the brain's inner components and the mental and physical cycles that these parts influence.

Calcium aids in the development of synapses and also helps in the formation of the framework through the mechanism by which they're released into the brain. The arrangement of Aloe's mineral is in line with the legitimate connection between mind and body.

Iron aids in the development of the sheath myelin fundamental which is responsible for the transmission of messages between cells and neurons. By the presence of iron, aloe only supports the proper functioning of this connection, but also helps to improve the health of blood vessels, which aids the cardiovascular system's efficient transfer of oxygen, blood, and other supplements to the brain.

Zinc is a crucial cerebrum health supplement provided by aloe to aid the cells involved in thinking, learning and memory, reducing the likelihood of developing degenerative conditions. It is believed to play a crucial role in the enzymatic processes which make control of muscles (both voluntary and mandatory) feasible but magnesium is just another mineral found in aloe

which works with the cerebrum's cycle and keeps up with the general wellbeing and the natural rhythms of the world.

Phytochemicals

In addition to providing the necessary supplements to support all the cycles associated by the mind Aloe has a variety of amazing phytochemicals that enhance the functioning of the cerebrum and safeguard its health. The cell-building substances in aloe aid in battling cell deformities that can lead to the development of diseases and block the the internal processes that the cerebrum performs. Antimicroscopic organisms and antiviral properties, aloe vera assists in reducing the risk of contamination in the cerebrum, by cleansing out blood (the conveyance framework which supplies the brain) and the cells of the cerebrum, as well as the an assortment of irresistible microbes, viruses, and bacteria.

One of the most beneficial benefits for maintaining the health of the cerebrum is its naturally occurring polysaccharides. Polysaccharides help in rehabilitating tissues and cells damaged by irritation, and also help to ensure the health of the existing tissues and cells that are responsible for every idea and activity which is controlled to the brain.

Recipes

Coconut Oil Coffee

The well-known mix of medium-chain unsaturated fats with coconut oil and an energized espresso, isn't just stimulating it is also beneficial to your body and mind as well.

Ingredients

Serves 2

12 ounces of hot fermented charged coffee

Half MUG ALOE VERA, JUICE

2 tablespoons coconut oil unadulterated

1. Blend espresso, aloe vera as well as coconut oil, in a mixer. Keep the opening opened to allow the hotness to release.

2. Blend until the espresso becomes foamy. It then changes to light brown.

3. Enjoy and drink!

Dark Cherry Dream

This purifying, want-to-control smoothie appears in a flash filled with nutrients and minerals to help to improve the functioning of the cerebrum.

Ingredients

Serves 2

1/4 CUP ALOE VERA JUICE

2 cups almond milk that is unsweetened, vanilla and unsweetened

1/2 cup pitted c herries

1/2 cup pitted dates

Half medium-sized banana de-stemmed and frozen

1 teaspoon ground cinnamon

Mix all the ingredients in the blender. Mix until smooth.

Great Guacamole

With powerful cancer-prevention ingredients that protect against sickness infections, infections, and the harmful changes to the body's cells, this delicious dip is a mind and body-soothing bite that you can enjoy any time.

Ingredients

Serves 2

1/4 CUP ALOE VERA JUICE

2 . Medium Hass avocados broken as well as pitted. 1 tablespoon lime juice

Half cup of diced red onions

1 cup chopped celery

1 cup chopped tomato

2 tablespoons lime juice

1. Mix avocados and aloe vera in a large bowl and squash until well-integrated but still chunky.

2. Mix in the remaining fixings and then toss using a fork until fixings are fully joined.

3. Refrigerate for up to two days. Cover with cling film that wraps around the entire face of the Guacamole, to prevent oxidization.

Banana-Nut Smoothie

This delicious blend of fixings is a great source of essential minerals, nutrients, and amino acids, while promoting mental health through the combination of antioxidants and omegas.

INGREDIENTS

SERVES 2

1/4 cup aloe vera juice

1/2 cup of cleaved walnuts

2 CUPPS NON SWEETENED VANILLA ALMOND MILK

1 MEDIUM BANANA, TRIPPED and FROZEN

1 teaspoon crushed cloves

1 teaspoon ground cinnamon

1. Combine pecans and aloe vera in a blender and blend on high until the pecans have blended.

2. Add the remaining fixings, then mix thoroughly until the fixings have been thoroughly mixed.

Completely combined.

Spicy Coffee Smoothie

Caffeine helps with intellectual work as well as concentration and thinking The naturally occurring phytochemicals offer protection against sickness in this delicious wake-up smoothie.

INGREDIENTS

SERVES 2

1/4 cup aloe vera juice

1 cup almond milk that is unsweetened, vanilla and unsweetened

11/2 cups of prepared stimulated espresso

Ground cayenne, chilled to 1/8th teaspoon

pepper

1 tablespoon natural maple syrup

Mix all the ingredients in blender. Mix until smooth.

Conclusion

This book is an easy and complete guide about aloe vera. It has briefly discussed about remarkable aloe vera plant, its uses, different methods of using aloe vera and its possible side effects. It has also guided you about planting your own aloe vera at home to get fresh aloe vera any time you want.

You can confidently use aloe vera for your own self and also for your family as it is safe for all. You will be surprised at seeing it's amazing results for health. You will find it friendly to your skin.

In this, book yummy recipes of several types of aloe vera drinks are also mentioned. You can try these at home. Also try aloe vera mask according to the type of your skin. You will notice that your skin will be ultra-soft and smooth. Sooner your friends and family will also notice a positive change in your skin. You can also suggest this book to your friends and family to let them know about this secret miracle healer plant.

I am pretty much sure that after reading this book there will be no question left unsolved about aloe vera, because this book provides a complete guideline about using aloe vera in different conditions.

Never forget key points while using aloe vera:

1.   In case of severe injury or infection do not go for a home remedy.

2.   If using aloe vera is not resulting in significant improvement then do not forget to consult your health care provider.

So start using aloe vera and enjoy its tremendous health benefits.